Praise for Looking Within

"**A memorable voyage into the mysteries of medicine.** The precision of a scientific mind, and the compassion of a true healer."

–Bob Rosen, best-selling author of *Conscious, Grounded, Leading People, Global Literacies,* and *The Healthy Company*

"**Dr. Cullen Ruff illuminates the breadth and power of medical imaging** as a diagnostic tool and goes beyond that to help us experience its beauty and poignancy, bringing the field, and the reader, out of the dark."

–Carolyn Jourdan, Wall Street Journal best-selling memoirist, biographer, and mystery writer.

"**Dr. Cullen Ruff sees through the images on the screen to the profound human stories they tell.** Compelling, compassionate, honest, and wise."

–Frank Huyler MD, author of *The Blood of Strangers, The Laws of Invisible Things,* and *Right of Thirst*

"**Compelling and insightful**—I urge everyone, physicians and the public alike, to read this brilliant work."

–James Borgstede MD, past president and chairman of the board of the American College of Radiology

"**A must read for patients and physicians alike.**"

– Susan Ascher MD, professor, Georgetown University School of Medicine

i

LOOKING WITHIN

*understanding ourselves
through human imaging*

LOOKING WITHIN

understanding ourselves
through human imaging

CULLEN RUFF

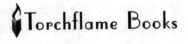
Torchflame Books

Durham, NC

Published 2020, by Torchflame Books
www.torchflamebooks.com
Durham, NC 27713 USA
SAN: 920-9298

Paperback ISBN: 978-1-61153-320-0
E-book ISBN: 978-1-61153-322-4
Library of Congress Control Number: 2019919061

The stories in this book are true and conveyed to the best of the author's recollection. Patient names have been changed or withheld. Information from colleagues was required for some chapters (e.g. "Abs of Steel" and "The Mule"). Partial descriptors were included for a former professor ("Self Discovery"); a former co-worker ("Yo-Yo"); and a current co-worker ("Family Secret") who has given permission to tell his story.

To teachers who have guided me, none more important than my parents, Carol F. Ruff, PhD and Judge Grady Ruff.

And to the many fine technologists with whom I have had the pleasure to work. Your knowledge, talents, and dedication are an inspiration, and a great service to the patients and doctors who depend on you.

Contents

IMAGES OF OURSELVES

My teachers in medical school were truly outstanding. One in particular, ironically named Dr. Biggers, exuded larger-than-life charisma, optimism, wit, and passion for his work, matched by his supersized girth. While giving our class a lecture one day on anatomy and disease of the head and neck, he showed slides of structures deep to the face, including the sinuses, pituitary gland, and nearby brain structures. Pointing to an area near the brainstem, a neurological junction of sorts where the brain meets the rest of the body—and where some of our most fundamental and essential functions like heartbeat and breathing are controlled—he made a barely audible comment: "And this is where the soul resides."

He said it on the sly, immediately proceeding to his next slide and continuing with his lecture. I am not sure how many other students even caught his statement, but I never forgot it. Dr. Biggers had a sense of humor, but he was also skilled at challenging students to think. Perhaps his comment was all in jest, but it still made me wonder about the ever-intriguing connections of mind, body, and spirit. Dr. Biggers helped plant a seed that encouraged my quest for the discoveries and revelations that may arise from peering into the very components that compose us. Looking into our own anatomy reveals images of ourselves, literally and metaphorically.

How did we get the ability to look within ourselves, and what might we learn from doing so?

Throughout history until the late nineteenth century, the human body could not be seen internally without cutting someone open. This changed dramatically in 1895, when the German scientist Wilhelm Roentgen discovered during an experiment that a beam of high-energy radiation could pass through a person and expose film. Having no existing name for this wavelength range of ionizing radiation, he simply named them "x-rays". The first x-ray image ever made, in fact, was of his wife's hand, as she assisted him in his laboratory. Startled by seeing the bones of her hand in this manner—something no one else had ever done—she reportedly found the image upsetting, fearing that she had seen a premonition of her own death. (In fact, she lived over two decades more, to die an old woman.)

For the first time, doctors could see pictures of people's bones and internal organs, helping diagnose everything from fractures to pneumonia. X-ray technology was adopted quickly within the field of medicine, given its remarkable usefulness, and Roentgen was awarded the first Nobel prize in physics in 1901 for his discovery. With more accurate diagnoses came more appropriate treatments for the diseases that people could now see internally, sometimes detected before the patient even showed symptoms. As scientists perfected x-ray technology and expanded its use, the field of radiology was born, revolutionizing the practice of medicine.

For decades, medical imaging was limited to variations on x-ray studies. However, in the latter part of the twentieth century, radiology blossomed to encompass other technologies such as nuclear medicine, ultrasound, computed tomography (CT), magnetic resonance imaging (MRI), and positron emission tomography (PET)—studies that many of us have had, or will have at some point, but which were completely foreign and unfamiliar to most people only a generation ago. The practice of medicine today, certainly in technically developed countries, would be unimaginable without the use of radiology.

Yet despite the vastly improved medical knowledge and treatments of today, people of course still get sick and ultimately die. We recognize this as part of life. For centuries, scholars, healers, spiritual leaders, and patients alike have searched for insight to life through dealing with illness and death. Sickness is unwelcome and challenging, if not overwhelming, but it sometimes helps us learn how to live better in the present, while also poignantly reminding us of our own mortality.

The true stories in this collection give readers perspective on various encounters with illness. By reading of others' experiences

with disease and injury, we may gain knowledg
that enhances our own path. Nevertheless, one
how these tales differ from others that descri
sickness.

The difference is the perspective from whic
disease, and the unique set of insights that has r
radiologist, a doctor who specializes in interpret
image the human body. The intriguing part of being   who
looks inside of people, at least indirectly, goes beyond the amazing
medical diagnostic potential of modern imaging; sometimes we
might find more than just a disease or condition. Occasionally
something unsuspected is detected. The discovery may be
something physical, or it may be intangible: something that tells a
story, makes us think, or teaches us something about people.

Unlike doctors who directly examine and consult with their
patients, I read studies of people whose primary doctors send them
for tests. I never even meet the majority of these patients, yet I
end up getting an intimate look inside their body parts. Sometimes
an expected abnormality is found, such as an injury, an infection,
a blood clot, or a tumor. Sometimes I find nothing wrong, to the
relief of everyone—particularly the patient, but also the patient's
doctor, and myself. Occasionally, I find something serious that was
not suspected by patients or their doctors.

When a discovery is made on an imaging study, radiologists
may find ourselves in the unique situation of being the first to have
special and intimate knowledge about the person being scanned.
At times this experience can be like glimpsing into the patient's
past or potential future, like looking into a crystal ball. We may
find something that could affect the person forever, like a tumor, a
stroke, or a fetus *in utero.* We may find something that will impact
the individual intensely in the short term, such as kidney stones
or appendicitis. We may see signs of an old injury or operation
that tells an interesting story about the person being studied. The
insight is obviously enhanced when we get to meet the patient
directly, but often the images alone tell us plenty.

Even beyond anatomy and disease, pictures of our inner
selves are worth way more than a thousand words. I do not just

eering beneath the adornment of our clothes, jewelry, oos, makeup, and scars. We can look much deeper than that. -rays, ultrasound, and magnetic fields cut through the surface like nothing else can. I believe that radiology can show us a completely different way of looking at people altogether, removing our superficial distinctions. Demographic information may be available in the medical records, but images themselves show no indication of someone's ethnicity, language, education, religion, attractions, wealth, or personality. Skin color, for example? No clue. I simply cannot tell.

There are obvious differences between the pediatric and the geriatric, but not for every organ; and for the majority of people between these extremes on life's spectrum, the distinctions of age are not always obvious. Gender is important to consider when looking for uterine or prostate cancer, but unless I am looking at certain specific body parts, it is often surprisingly easy to forget, or ignore, whether someone is even male or female. A heart is a heart; a brain is a brain.

Imaging is the great equalizer. When we look deep into ourselves from the vantage of this fundamental level, with exterior barriers and labels removed, we just might just see ourselves, other people, and our lives in a whole new light.

These unique aspects of looking into people have motivated me to write this collection of experiences. Examining people by looking within them can be fascinating, humbling, or awe inspiring, even to someone who has done this work for years. These feelings are part of what I hope to convey through recounting these patients' stories of medical imaging. Some of these stories inevitably have elements of sadness; others may contain surprise, hope, or even occasional humor. All are part of the emotional gamut that helps make life full.

As I reflect on these patients, and my brief but important relationship to them, I have found myself revisiting parts of my own education and development during medical school, internship, residency, fellowship training, and later into practice. Like everyone else's journeys, the process is ongoing. Most of us desire to be better tomorrow than we were yesterday, and doctors are certainly no exception. The approach of studying people from the inside out may be somewhat unique, but the process of looking within metaphorically still serves as a chance to learn, to appreciate, and to understand. Regardless of our experiences doing whatever each of us does, we all remain on a learning curve. We understand that everyone makes mistakes, including at work. I have included a few of my own mistakes here, partly because they were educational for me, and because they may be so for others as well. Ultimately, this book is simply about being human.

Since I began writing these stories to capture the personal elements of medical imaging with real-life vignettes, some of the personal touch has ironically been disappearing from the field, in the name of progress and productivity. Digital imaging and computerized report dictation have made our work faster and more efficient, allowing us to serve more people. However, having images and results more immediately available remotely has also decreased the personal interactions between doctors, other medical staff, and the patients we serve. Artificial intelligence is poised to become a larger and more integrated component of medical imaging, with people someday going under the knife because a computer algorithm diagnoses their appendicitis or breast cancer. Doctors behind the scene will definitely not disappear, but we may become even less visible. Stories of medical imaging, and of the radiologists and technologists who so directly impact patient care, need to be shared—even if we are sometimes as hidden as the illnesses we help discover in people.

Furthermore, as doctors and patients alike learn more about our health and the trajectories of our lives, we have to acknowledge, and accept, that our physical bodies have a yet-to-be-determined expiration date. This does not necessarily mean that our bodies ultimately fail us; perhaps they merely serve their purpose.

The art of looking into people holds amazing opportunities for observation, appreciation, and wisdom. May these stories and reflections inspire readers to live lives as healthy and whole as possible.

—Cullen Ruff MD

SECTION I:
GETTING STARTED

H aving graduated from medical school over twenty-seven years ago at the time of publication, I have seen hundreds of thousands of patients' studies of one kind or another. With most studies come multiple pictures, putting the number of medical images I have seen into the millions. Inevitably some cases are more memorable than others, but not necessarily more important, and the studies can be as unique as the subjects imaged.

Out of this very large pool, I begin with just a few cases that help illustrate the power of imaging. These stories may highlight the strength and resilience that people sometimes find within themselves, while simultaneously demonstrating the ultimate fragility of people, and of life itself. In these examples, we see different people from different walks of life, one of the perpetually interesting bonuses of working in medicine. In briefly studying these individuals, our perspectives are enhanced and enriched. We are all different people, but we may be more alike than we think.

HOLDING OUT

After two years of intense studies in classrooms and laboratories, many late nights, and the necessary memorization of unbelievable volumes of information, the students in my medical school class advanced to the patient wards for our third year of medical school. On a weekday August afternoon in 1990, I had just finished seeing all of the patients I followed, under the supervision of the residents and attending medical professor. The chief resident, a stocky fellow born in India, saw me in the hallway.

"Hey, which one of you medical students is on call tonight?" he asked.

"I am."

"Good. I just got a call about a patient who is being sent over from the clinic for admission to the hospital. She's a woman in her late thirties who had breast cancer several years ago. Now her doctor believes that she has a new lung cancer. That's an unusual history, to have two cancers by that age. It should be an interesting case."

I met the woman later that day, spoke with her about her medical history, and examined her before she was assigned a hospital room. "Mrs. A" was southern, very large, very talkative, and very nice. She joked about her unlucky medical history, trying to distract herself from worry by filling the room with honest but idle chatter. She was neither well educated nor shy. I liked her immediately.

"I just read the notes that your doctor sent over for us," I started. "I understand that you saw him for shoulder pain."

"Ouch, you better believe it!" she winced as she barely rotated her shoulder. "It's been getting worse for weeks now, and I haven't found *nothing* to make it better. I told my husband I'd finally get it checked out if y'all promise not to treat me like a horse and shoot me!" she winked.

"We won't even consider that," I smiled. "With my stethoscope and reflex hammer taking up so much space in this coat pocket, I've got no room for a pistol."

"Good!" she laughed. She had brought her shoulder x-ray films with her, and I held one up to the light. Since my ability to read films was nearly nonexistent then, it was fortunate that the radiologist had drawn erasable red crayon marks at the abnormal areas on the film, making it easy to find the abnormalities. Although the shoulder itself looked fine, there was a rather large mass in her left lung, near the center of her chest. Also labeled on the film was a lesion destroying part of a rib.

"What did your doctor tell you about these x-rays you had taken?" I asked.

"Well, he explained that, of all things, I've got a tumor in my lung! How's that for an unexpected surprise? And here I wondered if I must have pulled a muscle cleaning the house. I quit smoking several years ago. Don't know why I even started, to be honest, I was just young and stupid, trying to be cool and grownup like everybody else. I'd hate to add up what I spent on a pack a day for fifteen years. Well, I should have quit sooner, but I reckon it's still a good thing I quit when I did."

We continued by reviewing her history of breast cancer a few years beforehand. After feeling a breast lump that turned out to be cancerous, she had undergone a mastectomy and received some chemotherapy after the surgery.

"To think that after all I went through then, losing a breast and all, that I may have lung cancer now, all over again. Well, I just can't believe it. I still don't believe it. I guess cancer just loves my body," she said helplessly, raising her hands in the air.

I also was surprised, but for different reasons. She was younger, and had less of a cumulative smoking history, than most people with lung cancer.

"So I'm willing to come into the hospital if you all can figure out what to do for me," she said. "Hope you don't have to take out my lung, I'm already lopsided enough as it is!"

Later I presented the case to the intern on our team, a young man originally from Korea who had finished medical school in another state only two months prior. He agreed that we could not be sure whether this was a new lung cancer, as suspected by the clinic doctor, or in fact a breast cancer recurrence. Whichever it was, Mrs. A's long-term prognosis was guarded. The woman also had the rib lesion, which was highly suspicious for a metastasis. Whether from lung or breast cancer, the rib lesion meant that cancer had spread through her bloodstream and lodged in the bone. Since tumor had metastasized to that rib, it would likely spread to other sites as well, if it had not already.

The next morning at rounds, I presented Mrs. A's story to the other members of the internal medicine team, including the attending physician in charge, a friendly former New Yorker with graying hair. Because the x-ray film showed only one dominant lung mass, the professor and chief resident both believed that the woman probably had a new primary lung cancer. The intern had doubts, though, and recommended getting a tissue sample to confirm the diagnosis. However, the professor was not sure how easy it would be to biopsy the mass deep in her chest, or the diseased rib. I listened to the points made by my hierarchy of medical instructors, who politely countered each other without getting any closer to reaching a consensus on her condition. The discussion left me feeling slightly confused, no smarter, and a bit helpless.

After discussing our patients in the private conference room, the medical team made rounds together. I introduced Mrs. A to the rest of the doctors whom she had not yet met.

"Wow, with this many doctors, surely you all can come up with something that can nip this in the bud! Take your time. I'm counting on you all—you know where to find me!" she teased.

The intern asked me to obtain the written reports from the time of Mrs. A's mastectomy and the pathology records detailing the analysis of the tumor removed. The pathology report revealed that the patient's breast cancer at the time of mastectomy was big enough to be considered a stage III out of IV, despite the encouraging fact that none of the lymph nodes removed from her armpit had shown any cancer spread. She had received chemotherapy shortly after her surgery but had not seen an oncologist or taken prescribed medication for over two years. Whether or not she had been told so by a doctor, Mrs. A had assumed until recently that her cancer had been cured.

I checked on her late that afternoon. She had two visitors.

"Come on in here!" she beckoned, treating me as if I were a neighbor coming to call. "I want you to meet my husband and my oldest daughter. She knows she's my pride and joy." She turned to them. "He looks too young to be a doctor, don't he? I guess the rest of the doctors are a little bit older, but most of you all still look awfully young to me."

Although she masked any outward concern over her situation, the other family members spoke less and looked more worried. The husband was the most quiet, the stoic member of the family. The teenager asked a few relevant questions about her mother's condition and her pain control, exhibiting a surprising degree of responsibility and maturity.

"We thank you for your patience as we try to figure out what's going on here," I told them. "Sometimes cases are a bit confusing or complicated, but the doctors I'm working with are trying to figure out what these tumors are and how best to treat them."

Mrs. A jokingly interrupted. "They know if it involves me, it's rarely easy."

The teenage girl rolled her eyes and half-smiled, but the gesture did not conceal the concern on her face. "We just appreciate whatever you can do for her," she said. "We can be patient as long as it takes." The husband had been seated, staring at the floor, but he rose to shake my hand and thank me.

Another day passed. Nothing had really changed for Mrs. A, other than she had been started on mild narcotics for her pain, which had improved but not disappeared. I checked on her before morning rounds. She calmly rested in her bed and continued to amuse me during our conversations.

"I enjoyed meeting your husband and daughter yesterday. She seems like a dependable girl," I said.

"She's been a doll. She's rarely if ever given me any trouble.

She's really a big help with the younger children. With me being here in the hospital, she's doing all the cooking at home every day after school. My six-year-old twins in particular of course can't help do much at home, but they know I'm crazy about them, too. And while I'm stuck with this awful hospital food, maybe I'll finally lose a few of these extra pounds I'm carrying!"

Mrs. A seemed to trust that her doctors were trying to figure out her case in order to help her feel better. She never demanded that we rush to any judgment or opinion. We had no real news for her later that morning when the medical team came by to see her, but the medical professor did at least decisively determine the source of her shoulder pain. He pressed on her diseased rib during morning rounds, compressing the region of the partially destroyed area seen on the x-ray film. The wailing reaction that followed left no doubt that the rib lesion was causing the pain that radiated to her shoulder.

No progress was made, however, in reaching a consensus as to whether she had a new lung cancer or metastatic breast cancer. The team doctors decided to consult with a hospital oncologist.

That afternoon the oncologist met the patient and reviewed her chart, including the pathology report from the mastectomy. A white-haired man who looked old enough to retire, he pored over the woman's papers through his bifocals and never even entertained any diagnosis other than metastatic breast cancer. "I wouldn't give lung cancer another thought," he confided in me while writing a note in the patient's chart at the nurses' station. "I doubt we'll be able to do much for her long-term, but there are a couple of chemotherapy agents that apparently weren't used on her before. We could try a course of those and see how she does." He also switched her pain medicine to morphine, which did provide better relief.

At morning rounds the next day, I related to the rest of the team that the oncologist thought our patient had recurrent breast cancer, not lung cancer. The internal medicine professor was displeased. "Her diagnosis clearly *could* be metastatic breast cancer," he explained, "but we cannot jump to that conclusion. I certainly don't feel comfortable giving her chemo without knowing for sure what we're treating."

That afternoon, a special grand rounds was held. Multiple teams of specialists, residents, interns, and medical students attended to discuss several interesting cases, including Mrs. A, our friendly, talkative patient with the lung mass, rib lesion, and the previous breast cancer. The young Korean intern presented the woman's case history, after which the oncologist stood up in front of the gathering.

"I have reviewed her information," he began, "and would recommend a trial of chemotherapeutic agents she did not receive with her prior treatment a few years ago."

The internal medicine professor stood up and interrupted the oncologist. "We appreciate your reviewing this patient's case, but I have some concerns here in assuming a diagnosis of metastatic breast cancer rather than lung cancer, as was raised in the initial presentation."

"I believe that all of the evidence clearly points to recurrent breast cancer in her case," the oncologist stated firmly, holding his ground.

"I'm not saying that she doesn't have recurrent cancer," continued the internist, "I'm just saying that we need to be careful in making assumptions, particularly before prescribing chemotherapy."

The young intern spoke. "We really should have tissue diagnosis. I wish this could be more easily done than by removing a section of her rib."

"That would be preferable to cracking open her chest to resect that lung mass," said another doctor in the audience.

The mildly heated discussion continued. Everyone involved in the case wanted the patient to get the most accurate diagnosis and best treatment available, yet despite the more than one hundred years of combined medical experience in the room, there was difficulty reaching a consensus. As a student, I sat back and watched the mental sparring like a tennis match, uncertain as ever, not knowing what to think or whose opinion to value most. Finally, someone suggested that a CT scan be ordered to gather more information, and the parties involved agreed that the information from the scan might help solve the dilemma.

Again, the year was 1990, and we were at a university-affiliated regional hospital with a fine reputation. In retrospect, it amazes me that it took so long for the doctors to order the CT scan. Today most cancer patients routinely get periodic CT scans on an outpatient basis for at least several years, without ever being admitted to a hospital. CT could also be used to biopsy a mass, guiding the placement of a thin needle, without subjecting the patient to a more invasive surgery.

Mrs. A readily complied with the recommended CT scan. She drank the white barium solution, lay still on the scanner table, and received an iodine-based contrast injection into an arm vein, while x-ray beams passed through cross-sections of her head, chest, abdomen, and pelvis, one thin slice at a time.

I checked the scan results after dinner that evening. The radiologist was reading Mrs. A's study when I entered the dark reading room. He was studying several sheets of CT films hanging on the fluorescent view boxes in front of him.

"I'm sorry to interrupt while you're still reading her study," I apologized. "It's just that there has been some confusion regarding her diagnosis. She had breast cancer a few years ago, and now has a new lesion in her lung and her rib."

His tone was heavy. "Unfortunately, she's got a whole lot more than that. She's got metastatic cancer all over the place."

He pointed out the abnormalities on the films. The CT scan showed the main lung mass we knew about, but also other lung metastases too small to be seen on the regular chest x-ray. The lesion in her rib was visible, but the scan also revealed other bone metastases elsewhere that had not yet caused her any pain. The tumor had also spread to her liver and her brain.

I was devastated. This friendly, patient, slightly kooky woman would soon learn from this scan that she indeed had metastatic breast cancer throughout her body, despite the surgery and chemotherapy she had undergone a few years earlier. Her body held many hidden tumors giving her no symptoms yet. Eventually she could expect more pain, more debilitation, and essentially no hope for cure.

We solemnly broke the news to Mrs. A during rounds the next morning. The head professor briefly explained the CT findings while we stood alongside him, all of us facing her like an impenetrable wall. "The scan showed a number of other small tumors that we could not see on your x-rays," he began, detailing the lesions throughout her organs. "If a biopsy is needed for chemo, there is a spot in your liver that should be easy to sample, but the oncologist may not even require it. We now think that this is all coming from your breast cancer."

Mrs. A sat up in bed abruptly, stared at the internist, and said nothing. Her jaw dropped, her eyes opened wide, and her face silently spoke of disbelief and fear. She lay back down onto her side, looked away from us, and asked no questions at that time.

Finally, I realized why she had been able to make light of her situation until that moment. As long as she could maintain some uncertainty regarding the lung and rib tumors on her shoulder x-ray, she could hope, deny, or delay. Now that she had enough information to grasp the seriousness of her illness, her mind would no longer allow her to escape. She could no longer distract herself from thinking about what this news meant for her and for her family. Breast cancer was scattered throughout her body. The surgery and chemotherapy a few years before had not cured her after all, and she had every reason to believe now that nothing could.

Mrs. A remained in the hospital for a few more days, and she remained despondent much of the time. A couple of days later, however, she was a bit more animated when I checked on her in the early morning.

"My sister's coming to see me today," she announced.

"Oh, really. You haven't mentioned her before. What's she like?" I asked, wondering if she had as much personality as this patient of whom I was so fond.

"She's *fat!*" she blurted.

It was an odd statement, but accurate: her sister was obese, although not nearly so much as Mrs. A herself. Our team of doctors happened to meet her sister later that morning during rounds. We spoke with Mrs. A, asking how she was feeling that day, while her sister listened by the bedside. As we left the room, the sister followed us out into the hallway. Mrs. A leaned forward and watched with keen interest from her bed, eyeing us until we were beyond the closed door.

"I didn't want to ask you all in front of her," the sister began, "but how long does she have to live?"

"That's difficult to say," began the doctor in charge of the team. "It depends on a lot of things. Ultimately she will die from this, but when, that's hard to predict right now."

"OK," she said, while I wondered more about the sisters' relationship.

"By the way," he asked her, "have you had a mammogram?"

"No," she said, sounding disappointed in herself for having procrastinated so long.

"You need to get one," he advised.

Later that day I checked on Mrs. A once more. She was mildly upset.

"What did my sister ask you all today in the hall?" Her tone strengthened my suspicion that their relationship, like those of many relatives, was a bit complicated.

I did not want to hurt her feelings. I did not want her to be further upset, or to have to face any more negative thoughts than she already had that day. "She asked about your treatment, and how long you might be in the hospital," I said, trying to dodge the question.

Her face revealed an expression she had not shown throughout her hospitalization. The answer did not satisfy her. She knew instinctively that I had not told her the truth. Already she could no longer trust her body, her previous treatment, perhaps even her faith. Now she had reason not to trust me.

It took a few days to get back to our earlier rapport, but we did. The experience taught me that she deserved the truth like everybody else. She may not have expected a perfect cure, but she had every right to honesty. Since then, there have been many, many times that I have broken bad news or answered other uncomfortable questions. Sometimes people want it straight up, delivered bluntly and directly. Other times, the situation or personalities may require a gradual divulgence, occasionally soft pedaling or sugarcoating, to allow people time to process information they need but definitely do not want. We do the best we can in each situation, but I can honestly say that I have never lied to a patient since.

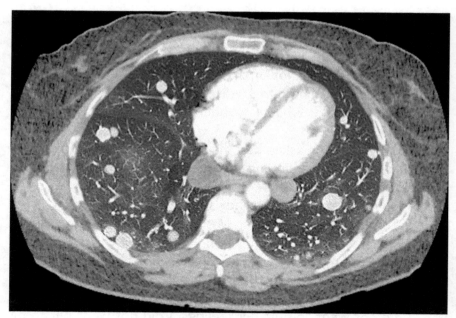

Breast cancer metastases to lung
A cross-section image of a chest CT. The small round lesions are lung metastases. (The large central structure is the heart.)

I visited Mrs. A regularly until she was discharged. Even when she considered me her ally again, our interactions were understandably less animated as her condition deteriorated. Given her young age, and the fact that she had children at home, she was leaning toward trying whatever treatments might be available, and we tried to be positive about benefits she might receive from future chemotherapy or radiation. Still, the conversations were stifled. She was more often detached, deep in thought, or sometimes trying to get reacquainted with her Bible.

After all of the academic discussion and differences of opinion that had preceded, one CT scan answered the question that had perplexed some of her doctors for days. The results also confirmed the woman's unfortunate fate. As a medical student, I was amazed by the informative power of one CT scan, which put to rest all of the academic discussion and uncertainty of her diagnosis up to that point. Yet, I was also left feeling saddened and fairly helpless by the information it revealed. I had learned a lesson in how technology may help make a diagnosis, but I recognized that in her case, the outcome would be the same. We all knew what she had now, but we did not know how to cure her. While we acknowledged our limits in treating her disease, we were devastatingly precise in its prognosis.

Mrs. A would have some time left ahead to live, and I hope that she made each day as meaningful as possible. Perhaps the limited treatments she received after that point provided her some extra quality time, or at least made her more comfortable. However, other than helping with pain management, and providing an occasional ear to listen, or a hand to hold, I fear that we ultimately offered her little more than a diagnosis.

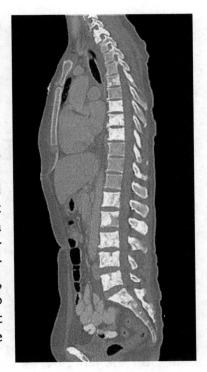

Above: Bone metastases. A lateral view from a CT scan. The white lesions within multiple vertebrae are skeletal metastases in a patient with breast cancer.
Below: Liver metastases. The round darker gray lesions represent breast cancer metastases in the liver.

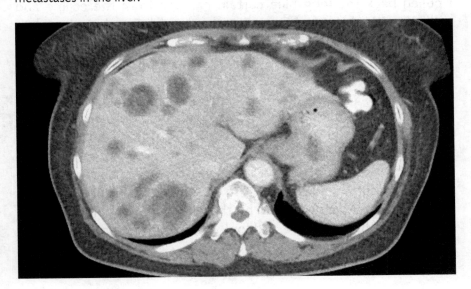

REVERSAL

Early in my internship, only a few months after graduation from medical school, I was on call one night at the hospital. It was a Thursday evening in the early Carolina fall, and the weather was still quite hot. Long after dark had set in, I got paged to the emergency room.

The physician running the emergency department motioned me over. "I've got a man for you to admit. He's a crack user who has had left-sided weakness since he was smoking several days ago. I think he suffered a stroke, with a significant motor and sensory deficit on the left side, as well as some visual loss. Mentally he's groggy, but he's fairly oriented and can give you a history. He just got back from CT, so they ought to have his scan result soon."

He pointed to the numbered cubicle where the patient lay. I pulled back the long blue curtain hanging from the ceiling and walked inside the space. On a stretcher lay a disheveled white man in his early thirties. He was alone. His Harley Davidson cap had been set aside, and his matted, long brown hair needed washing. His ragged beard was speckled with gray. A nurse had removed his soiled black T-shirt and faded blue jeans, and laid them to the side of the stretcher. He was lying still, wearing only a pair of dirty underwear, with his fleshy white belly protruding over the upper elastic. He looked dazed, as if he were sleeping with his eyes open.

I put my right hand in his, noticing the grime under his nails. I squeezed softly. "Hey there, I'm Dr. Ruff," I said, only recently accustomed to calling myself by that title. "We're going to bring you into the hospital here and look after you until you get better. What's your name?"

He hesitated, taking a moment to turn his head and meet my gaze. "Ronnie," he replied.

"Ronnie, can you tell me what happened?" I asked.

He spoke slowly and softly in a tired, raspy voice. "Yeah, I've been weak and feeling bad for several days. On Monday, the friend I'm staying with brought home some crack, and we smoked it. I hadn't done it too many times, but that time was different. When I woke up the next day, I was having trouble seeing, and trouble walking. My foot was dragging, and I was bumping into walls. My arm's also real weak, I can't lift nothing. I didn't feel good, and just laid on the couch the whole next day."

"You didn't see a doctor then," I confirmed, knowing the answer was *no* if he was just now coming to the emergency room.

"I was hoping I'd get better on my own."

"So what happened next?" I asked.

"Well, my friend had left the apartment the next morning, and didn't come home for a couple of days. I didn't have nobody else to call. I've got a wife, but we've been separated for a little while," he said.

I looked down at his large, dirty hands and saw no wedding ring.

"Does she live in the area?" I asked.

"Yeah, I saw her a couple of weeks ago. We're on OK terms, we've just got some issues and are taking a little break," he explained.

"OK, so fill me in on what happened next," I continued. "You realized you were having trouble seeing and walking, and that your arm was weak. When your symptoms didn't go away, what did you do next?"

"Nothing at first. I tried getting a hold of the guy I'm staying with, and I reached him Wednesday, yesterday. I told him I wasn't doing too good, but he said he was busy with something and couldn't come home until today," he said.

"You didn't think about calling an ambulance?" I asked.

"No, I just kept hoping this would go away," he said.

"So your friend finally did show up today?"

"Yeah, although he didn't bring me here. He brought some money and wanted me to go back out to get some more crack.

It took me awhile to walk down to where I get it, because I ain't moving well, but I did make it back there. But down at the spot, a young woman I've seen a couple of times starting talking to me, and noticed that I don't look too good. She went and got a friend of hers who has a car, and they brought me here."

"Are they still here?" I asked.

"No," he answered, "I thanked them and told them to go on home."

"Before this happened, what kind of shape were you in?" I asked. "Any medical problems?"

"No, I was just fine," he replied. "I was working sometimes as a roofer."

I proceeded to ask more questions, confirming that he was oriented to the date and to his surroundings. Although slow and somewhat listless, he answered questions appropriately. He even asked a few, although one in particular caught me off guard.

"I guess I won't have no trouble getting disability after this, will I?" he asked.

I hesitated, surprised by the question and its implications. "Let's just look after you, try to get you better, and hope you don't have to cross that bridge," I replied.

I examined him more thoroughly, particularly with regard to his neurological system. I held up two fingers in front of his face, watching his eyes follow my hand. I checked his reflexes, strength, and sensation, alternately lightly poking him with both the sharp and dull ends of my reflex hammer. Afterward, when I sat down to write his admission orders, the nurse tapped me on the shoulder.

"The radiologist is on the phone with your patient's CT result," she said.

I picked up the phone.

"I've got this fellow's CT in front of me," the doctor began. "Is there any chance he has been doing cocaine?"

"As a matter of fact, he has. He was smoking crack and has symptoms of a stroke. How did you know?" I asked.

"Because he's bled into his brain, and I don't see an aneurysm. Around here, someone his age with a CT like this is often a cocaine abuser. He's also got a little more brain atrophy than you would expect for somebody his age. He has probably been partying with one thing or another for a long time."

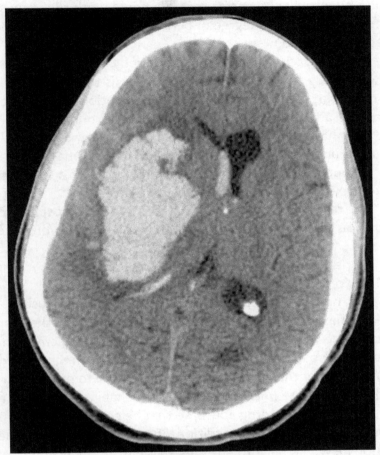

Hemorrhagic stroke
The large bright lesion in the right side of the patient's brain
on this head CT scan represents recent bleeding.

After finishing the written orders to get Ronnie admitted to the hospital, I went to look at his CT with the radiologist. Sure enough, there was a pool of fresh blood within the right side of his brain, accounting for the left-sided stroke that his body had just suffered a few days ago. The parts of the brain where blood had collected were in areas known to help control movement, sensation, and vision. The blood would get reabsorbed over time, but the areas of dead brain tissue would not regenerate. His residual network of living neural pathways might learn to help compensate for his physical limitations from the stroke, but some debilitation would undoubtedly be permanent. He could work to regain some lost functions, but the degree of permanent deficit would remain a mystery for a while.

I walked back and looked at him briefly. He had fallen asleep and was lightly snoring, his mouth agape. His teeth had not been well cared for, and he smelled. A drug prevention campaign could not ask for a better poster child. One mistake, one moment of an illicit high, had cost him some living brain tissue and rendered him with a yet undetermined amount of permanent damage.

I tapped on his right shoulder lightly. It took a moment for him to wake and respond with a dull, flat look.

"We're going to get you sent upstairs to a hospital room. Would you like me to call your wife and let her know you're here?" I asked.

He hesitated to answer. "She ain't got no phone."

"Anyone else then?" I asked.

"No, not right now," he slurred, his gaze still unfocused.

The next morning I presented this man's case to the team of doctors, who met him later that morning as we collectively made rounds on our patients. There was not much to do in the immediate aftermath, other than control his blood pressure to prevent further bleeding. The more important issue was rehabilitation, both from the stroke and for his drug abuse, so that he could recover as much as possible and prevent any additional future strokes. The domestic situation he would fall into after discharge from the hospital would be a key ingredient in the potential success of his recovery. This patient needed a whole lot more support than he had prior to coming into the hospital.

We met with a hospital social worker, a helpful and impressive woman. Confident but not pushy, she seemed intelligent and finessed. Her hair was blond and well cut, and she looked stylish in a colorful silk dress and pearl necklace. Her speech was measured and poised, but her manner was appropriately direct and to the point with Ronnie, who was clearly of a different socioeconomic class and educational level.

When the social worker and I sat down and talked with Ronnie, we learned that his past was quite checkered. Before moving in with his recent roommate, he had briefly stayed at a nearby homeless shelter. Ronnie had once served time in prison, and did not have a history of steady employment. He worked odd jobs, most recently as a subcontracted roofer on a construction site. He had no children.

We also came to understand that he had never been legally married. The woman he referred to as his wife earned that status by common law arrangement, the legal nuances being unfamiliar to me then.

The social worker presented the possible options for his placement after his eventual release from the hospital and stroke rehabilitation program. She summarized our discussion with him up to that point. "So, we're talking about two very different types of rehab. One is the rehab for the stroke you had. The other of course is the rehab for the drugs."

He nodded.

"We need to have some idea where you will live after you've finished with the rehab programs," she continued. "If your wife—what was her name?"

"Lori," he said.

"If Lori is willing to take you in and look after you, great. You'll need someone reliable so you can have a stable situation. However, I gather that you have some question as to whether or not you may be able to live with her again," she stated, being direct but empathetic.

"It's possible she don't want me back no more," he said. "I'll just have to tell her what happened and ask her."

"And what would you do if she says no?" I asked. "Is there someone else who could serve as a backup? A relative, or friend perhaps?"

"No, not really," he said. "The friend I was staying with last week sure didn't help me none."

The social worker and I looked at each other in silent agreement.

"Well," she continued, "let's talk to Lori first, and come up with an alternative plan if we need to." She had already determined that the man had no insurance or financial means for private care.

"There is a waiting list for the few halfway houses in the area, and the rules are fairly rigid there," she said. "We could always consider a homeless shelter if necessary."

He stared straight ahead, his face remaining nearly expressionless. "I'd rather go back to prison," he said dryly.

He had spent time in both jail and homeless shelters before. He knew exactly what he was talking about.

Ronnie remained in the hospital for a number of days, working with physical and occupational therapists, in order to regain some lost motor skills. I watched one therapist work with him, as Ronnie practiced picking up plastic poker chips with his weak hand and putting them into a paper cup. His steadiness was improving, but he clearly had a way to go. He spent a lot of time napping, and I was not sure how hard he was trying to recover at times, particularly when the application process for disability was underway. A man of few words, he was not outwardly thankful for our services, but neither did he complain or cause trouble. His expression remained dulled, and he still had some trouble focusing visually. One eye remained glassy and vacant.

To confirm that the bleeding had not worsened within Ronnie's brain, one of the residents ordered a follow-up CT scan a week later. There was no new hemorrhage. The old blood already spilled within his brain was beginning to degrade and would be reabsorbed by the surrounding tissue over time, leaving a vacant hole behind. As the stroke matured, Ronnie was learning to evolve. He would have to keep trying, while we waited to see how well he would recover.

Glad that he was making at least some progress, I was equally pleased when I saw the social worker in the hospital a few days later. She gave me the news that she had contacted the patient's common-law wife, and that the woman would take him back and aid with his recovery. Later that morning, I got a page from the hospital operator, who connected me to the young woman whom I had not yet met.

"Hi, this is Lori," she said over the telephone. Between

identifying herself by first name only, and her timid voice, she sounded a bit like a scared child talking to an authoritative adult. She relaxed when I thanked her for calling and told her that I was looking forward to meeting her. We both acknowledged being pleased that Ronnie was improving each day.

"That lady social worker told me that I needed to call you and let you know if I'm interested in having Ronnie move back in with me, to look after him when he's better. The answer is *yes*, I'm *very* interested," she said.

I did meet her at the hospital on a later date, before Ronnie was discharged. A small woman with flat, brown hair, she was no more sophisticated or articulate than Ronnie. She came across as passive and meek, and I feared she had the traits of someone who might easily be abused, or at least manipulated. I had no reason to assume this was happening, though, and just hoped that she was up for the challenge. The important thing was that she was willing to look after Ronnie. She at least seemed dutiful and committed, and she was by far his best option.

Eventually Ronnie was discharged and moved back in with Lori, avoiding both prison and the homeless shelter. He missed his clinic follow up appointment, and I did not see him for several months, until I was in the emergency room another night. Ronnie did not see me. He was walking back and forth between a secretary at the desk and a curtained off emergency room bed. I could not see the individual behind the curtain, but could hear a woman moaning and yelling obscenities. Ronnie lingered in the holding area with the agitated patient, obscured by the curtain. Periodically he would exit to get an update from the secretary and nurses at the desk. I particularly noticed him when he seemed pleased with their latest statements. He clapped his hands together enthusiastically, showing no sign of the shakiness or weakness that he had demonstrated several months ago.

"Okay then!" he said, turning back to check on the woman cursing and resisting behind the curtain. He had regained his ability to smile, quite satisfied with whatever the staff had just told him. I was close enough to see that one eye still looked glazed and unfocused, but he had no more trouble walking or speaking clearly.

A policeman stood outside of the patient's curtain. On the other side, the restrained woman continued screaming vulgarities. After Ronnie walked back behind the curtain, I approached the three women working at the desk.

"I treated that man a few months ago," I told them. "Who is that in there?"

"His girlfriend," one of the nurses said. "She's drunk as a skunk."

"Is her name Lori?" I asked.

"That's the one," the secretary confirmed. "She's in here all the time, raising hell after getting out of control like this. I don't know why these people keep coming here every time they go on a binge and get unruly. We don't do much for them."

"I can see why nobody else would want to put up with them though, and would call the cops just to get some peace and quiet," the second nurse said. "Still, all we do is restrain her and let her dry out."

"What was he happy to hear just now?" I asked.

"She fell and bumped her head before coming here, and we were waiting on her head CT. The radiologist just called and said it was normal, other than her not holding still. But no injury, so maybe they can drag her drunk ass out of here."

"Is he usually with her?" I asked.

"Oh yeah, they're a team," the secretary replied. "He may not be much of a catch, but I reckon she's lucky to have him."

PEOPLE LIKE US

On call another evening of internship, I was paged by one of the emergency room doctors. "We've got an admission to the medicine service. He's a young guy with AIDS who comes in with two days of worsening abdominal pain. His symptoms suggest appendicitis, except that he's got a normal white blood cell count. The surgical residents just finished seeing him and don't find any reason to operate, but I'm not comfortable sending this guy home. His symptoms and story are worrisome enough to me that we should at least observe him overnight."

The surgical residents were writing notes in the patient's chart when my chief resident and I entered the emergency room. The patient lay nearby behind the cubicle drape. The one female surgery resident in the program, whose short stature was overshadowed by her cockiness, greeted us with a barely concealed grin of victory.

"It looks like this one's yours," she said, "because we're not touching him."

"Let me take a look at him," I said. "You don't think he's got appendicitis, like the ER doc was thinking?"

"No way," she said.

"His white count is only six thousand," the tall male surgery resident with her said, referring to the body's white blood cells which increase when fighting an infection.

"Is that reliable in patients with AIDS?" I asked. "Depending on how immunocompromised he is, his baseline might be lower than that. Six thousand may be normal for you or me, but couldn't that be high for him, if he may usually run lower?"

"Be my guest to take a look at him," she said, "but we're not cutting him. He didn't even have that impressive of an exam. Look,

29

I'll show you myself."

She led the way into the man's cubicle. The patient was a lean but normally muscled man in his early thirties. His mullet-styled hair came to the bottom of his neck in the back, with short bangs in the front that spiked up, framing his tanned face. His teeth flashed white in contrast to his brown goatee, as he reached out to shake my hand.

"This is my mother." He gestured to a pleasant woman standing by his side. She was trying to mask her concern. I glanced back at the patient and privately agreed with the surgical residents' assessment: the man did not look noticeably sick.

We spoke for a moment about his symptoms. He began feeling poorly the day before he came to the emergency room.

"How bad is your pain right now?" I asked.

"It's pretty bad," he said. "It started out with just feeling queasy, with no appetite, but the pain has gotten worse all day and moved mostly down low on this side," he gestured toward his lower right abdomen.

"Let me feel your belly," I said, placing my hands on his abdomen. The skin and muscles were soft and accommodated my pressing on his right lower quadrant. He did flinch a bit when I suddenly released the pressure. The female surgeon repeated the move, and again the man winced briefly.

"It's going to take more than that to be considered rebound tenderness," she muttered to me as she exited the room.

"I promise you it hurts," he said. "I wouldn't be here if it didn't."

"No, I believe you," I said. "We want to bring you into the hospital so we can keep an eye on you and see how you do overnight. Do you still have your appendix?"

"Yes I do, I've never had surgery."

"Have you had any fever with this?"

"He's definitely warm," his mother spoke. "He often has a low grade fever, we presume on account of the AIDS." She spoke the words freely, and I was intrigued by her honesty and comfort level. Obviously honesty and comfort are important, and encouraged, when communicating to doctors, but AIDS was still a particularly delicate topic in 1993, despite its increasing prevalence.

On the surface, his mother looked like she could have been a matron of any of the small southern town's churches, some of which vocally condemned people with the deadly infection that still carries a stigma. Yet by speaking candidly, she revealed herself simply as a mother concerned for the health and well-being of her son. She was not ashamed to acknowledge that he had once contracted a virus that would not leave.

"I do often run a low-grade fever," he agreed, "but my temperature feels worse today."

We reviewed his medications, allergies, and medical history, which was not that involved for someone with his disease. He had not had any of the life-threatening infections or cancers that many AIDS patients eventually get.

After writing the orders to admit him to the hospital, I retrieved his old records later that evening. At that time in that hospital, medical records were hard copy and not digitized. Notes in patients' charts were mostly hand-written, with varying degrees of legibility. Even old lab tests were not always retrievable by computer, resulting in a delay of several hours before I could get the data necessary to assess his situation.

He definitely had AIDS by blood test criteria, namely that he was HIV positive and had a low T-cell count. Still, he had not yet suffered other serious AIDS complications. It was noteworthy, however, that his white blood cell count several months before was low at 2300, due to the virus's effects in weakening his immune system. His current level of 6000 would be normal for a healthy person, but was more than double his most recent baseline level. Odds were that had an acute infection somewhere in his body, presumably where he hurt.

AIDS was powerful at that time for so many reasons. It had already killed many people, often individuals who were young and previously healthy. AIDS also forced people to confront uncomfortable social and personal issues that were often avoided or denied, primarily people's sexuality. Although there were a number of folks in that small town with the disease, people with AIDS were often viewed with suspicion, even by some hospital employees who were paid to treat them. Part of that was an understandable genuine fear. Any health care worker suffering an accidental needle stick might end up contracting the nearly universally fatal disease, with few treatment options.

Yet part of the wariness was of the people themselves, rather than the disease they had. Having cared for other AIDS patients that year, I knew that the disease disproportionately affected those with marginal social positions, including gays, low-income blacks, and drug addicts. Having AIDS was yet another reason for some people who already faced challenges in life to be looked down upon by others.

On one occasion a nurse referred to one of my female patients with AIDS as "one of the innocent ones." I said nothing to the nurse at the time, but I remember thinking that the patient had contracted the virus by having unprotected intercourse, like most of the male AIDS patients. Yet in the nurse's eyes the woman was somehow sanctified, while the gay men in particular were vilified.

Early the next morning I checked on my current patient before rounds, apologizing for waking him. He responded that he had not rested well anyway.

"How are you feeling today?"

"Worse," he said. His fever had spiked overnight, and his abdomen hurt more, so much that it pained him to shift position while lying in bed. He looked weaker. His white cell count had risen to 8100, still normal for a healthy person but suspiciously climbing for him.

At morning rounds we presented the man's case to our professor, who went with us to examine the patient. The young man's abdomen at that point was distended and taut, much more tender than it had been the day before. Now he really looked sick.

"Of course, in his case, the culprit could be a number of things, including opportunistic infections, even lymphoma," the attending physician agreed as we spoke afterward outside the patient's door. "But I'd sure keep appendicitis in the differential. The surgeons need to see him again this morning."

"I'll make sure they do, but they're going to need more convincing," I said. "It's understandable. I wouldn't want to risk exposing myself either. But he's got something acute, and his AIDS is not end-stage. He was working and feeling good only a few days ago."

"We could always get a CT scan in his case, given the different possibilities, if that might shed some light," he suggested.

The CT scan was done later that day. The radiologist called to let us know that the man did indeed have appendicitis. Our team of doctors and medical students went to review the scan, which showed a dilated and inflamed appendix.

"Any sign of rupture?" we asked.

"No," the radiologist cautioned, "not yet."

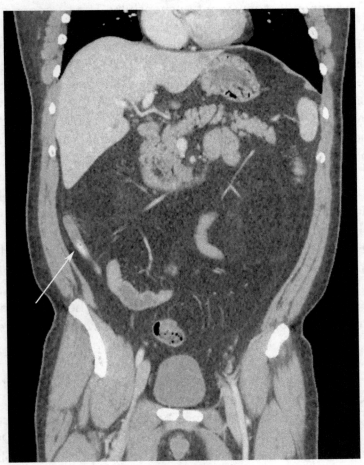

Appendicitis
Coronal view in a CT scan demonstrating an inflamed,
fluid filled appendix consistent with appendicitis.

On hearing the news, the surgeons also reviewed the CT with the radiologist, then became resigned to operate. Both surgeons who had been so outspoken the day before were considerably quieter, having been proven wrong. They no longer protested the diagnosis. Understandably, they were still nervous to operate, in fear for their own safety. There was only one anti-retroviral medication available at that time to combat HIV, a drug called azidothymidine, or AZT. At best, it slowed the virus's progression. It was definitely no cure. One mishap in the operating room, and an unintended exposure might mean an eventual death sentence for a surgeon.

The appendectomy went uneventfully. The surgeons did not cut or puncture themselves during the operation.

The patient improved each day after surgery, and his mother was visibly delighted when I found her visiting him two days later. "We're just so pleased with his progress," she said as he sat up in bed, smiling at both of us. "I was afraid that his recovery would be slower than usual, but I've known other people who had their appendix removed, and he seems to be coming along as fast as anybody else."

"He has done well. It looks like you're going home tomorrow," I said, shaking his hand at first, then spontaneously briefly placing my hand on his head, tousling his hair for just a second like a kid at school might do. That brought him his first smile in several days.

He left the hospital feeling stronger, and he followed up a few days later with the surgeons in their clinic, returning to work the following week. After his recovery, his baseline white blood cell count dropped to 1500, one-fourth the level he had on the day he came to the hospital. His immune system was steadily getting worse, but for the time being, he was hanging on as best as he could.

His recovery from the appendicitis was rapid. His longer term prognosis was still considerably more guarded.

Timing may be everything, however, as medical research paved the way to new discoveries and developments. Only a couple of years later, antiviral drugs called protease inhibitors became available, and many people with HIV, even those with fairly advanced disease, saw dramatic improvements in their immune function and overall health. People taking the newer drugs could live considerably healthier lives. I saw some patients rebound amazingly, even returning to work after AIDS had left them temporarily disabled. These people could live independently again, with markedly prolonged life expectancy. As a bonus, the people taking medication to minimize their own viral loads became much less likely to infect others.

If this man lived just two or three years more, long enough to receive protease inhibitors, there is a decent chance that he might still be alive today. I don't know whether he is or not. I finished internship a few months after meeting him in the hospital, and then moved far away to start residency.

But I do still remember the day he left the hospital. His nurse called me, letting me know that the man had left something behind with my name on it. I stopped by the nurses' station to find a vase with a red rose, one that someone else had sent him as a get-well wish. I opened the makeshift note card and read his one-word inscription to me.

"Thanks."

Editorial comment: Historically, many patients with symptoms of appendicitis underwent surgery solely based on their presentation, symptoms, physical exam, and lab tests. Today where imaging is available, however, just about everybody with symptoms of appendicitis gets an imaging study to confirm the diagnosis before undergoing surgery. (CT is most commonly used. For pregnant women and some children, MRI or ultrasound is used, as these studies, although not quite as sensitive as CT, emit no radiation, something particularly desirable in children and pregnant women.) In prior years it was acceptable that a fairly high percentage of appendectomies removed an appendix that was actually normal. Imaging today spares people the risk, expense, hospitalization, and recovery time of unnecessary surgery.

DETECTIVE WORK

After medical school and internship, I began radiology residency, moving over halfway across the country to the city I would call home for the next four years. The other residents and I worked apprentice-style with our professors who taught us their specialty. It did not take long to realize how difficult the learning process could often be. It also soon became apparent that sometimes the most subtle findings can have the greatest significance.

I began the first month by learning to perform gastrointestinal barium studies. The patients drank heavy, white metallic liquid before lying down on the x-ray table. They were then instructed to roll into different positions while the x-ray tech and I took pictures of their esophagus, stomach, and small intestine, the "upper GI" tract. Less pleasant for patients were barium enema studies to evaluate the colon.

Only one week into my residency training, I was reading cases with my professor, a bespectacled man who looked academic in his long white coat. Suzanne, a young radiologist new to the department, came to visit him. She also wore a white coat, looking professional. A small woman with wavy blond hair pulled into a ponytail, she seemed outgoing, confident but friendly. Suzanne had just finished her residency out of state and had recently passed her radiology board examinations.

"I don't know if you remember meeting last week at orientation," she reintroduced herself. "I'm one of the new abdominal imaging fellows."

"Of course, I remember you," he nodded. "What can we do for you?"

"I'd like you both to look at this x-ray, to confirm what I am afraid I'm seeing. I was asked to do a portable ultrasound of this woman's abdomen. It was the first study that I've done by myself since starting here last week, and I wanted to make a good first impression."

"I respect that," he smiled.

"Well, I ran into a big problem," she continued. "It was one of the hardest and worst studies I've ever done. There's nothing wrong with the ultrasound machine, but my images were awful. The woman came into the hospital yesterday with dehydration, low blood pressure, and shortness of breath. She's gotten much worse since she arrived and is now unconscious. They had to put her on a ventilator. Meanwhile, her abdomen has become more distended, and her doctors asked us to scan her."

"So what did you see?" he asked.

"I couldn't see anything," she replied. "Her abdomen was just full of gas, blocking everything and making it a really horrible study. Before I went to show the other ultrasound folks how bad these images looked, I came to look at her x-ray films, to make sure there wasn't some explanation."

Suzanne hung a single chest x-ray film in front of us on the view box. One week into my residency, I saw nothing wrong.

"She hasn't had any abdominal films taken, but this is her chest x-ray from this morning," she continued. "It was read as basically normal."

I could practically see the cogs turning in his head as the professor studied the x-ray. "It was read as normal? I hope I'm not the one who read this," he joked dryly.

"No, it was somebody else," she assured him. "And I think he was right about the chest, but it's the upper abdomen I'm worried about. Look at her liver. Doesn't that look like portal venous gas?"

Suzanne pointed to the patient's liver, just below the right lung, and she outlined slightly darkened areas that resembled the shape of a branching tree.

"It sure does," he agreed, then turned to me. "Pay attention, Cullen, you are about to learn something."

"Once you've seen this, you'll remember it," she said to me. "She's probably infarcted a lot of bowel, and if so, she's probably going to die soon."

I had never seen this abnormality before, and that was a fortunate thing, because patients with gas in the veins to the liver are usually critically ill, if not mortally so. The problem is not so much the gas in those veins, but what caused the gas to get there in the first place.

In this elderly smoker, blocked arteries and severe dehydration resulted in poor circulation to her intestines, impairing the blood supply to her bowel so badly that the tissue did not receive enough oxygen to stay alive. Portions of her intestines had recently died due to inadequate blood supply, and gas had broken through the intestinal walls to the veins that drain the blood from her bowel to her liver. There the gas had lodged in some of the vein branches of her liver, causing the telltale sign of impending death on the x-ray film.

The radiologist who read the chest x-ray that morning had been right regarding his interpretation of the chest, but by far the most important finding on that film was not even in the chest, but in the upper abdomen. He had missed a "corner finding," an abnormality seen only near the edge of a film. When people look at a picture—whether a photograph, a painting, or an x-ray image— our gazes are usually naturally drawn to the center. A detective analyzing photographs, or a radiologist reading x-rays, learns to examine everything on the entire image, even though this exercise is contrary to human nature and requires continual discipline. Sometimes the subtle, peripheral findings may reveal the greatest information, provided that one looks for these clues in the first place.

Reassured that she was not imagining the drastic x-ray findings, Suzanne immediately called one of the doctors in the intensive care unit and broke the news.

"Are you sure?" he asked.

"I'm afraid so," she said almost apologetically. "You could always get a quick abdominal film if you want to confirm and see the rest of her intestines."

"We will immediately," he assured her. "I'm afraid you're going to be right. It would explain a lot, because she's really going downhill."

The abdominal x-ray showed more gas within the liver and in the walls of dilated intestinal loops throughout her abdomen.

"I don't guess there's anything they can do at this point?" I asked my professor.

"I don't think so," he shook his head. "I doubt she was a strong candidate for surgery to begin with, but when this much intestine is gone, it's generally too late even to try to restore any blood supply. I'm afraid she's not long for this world."

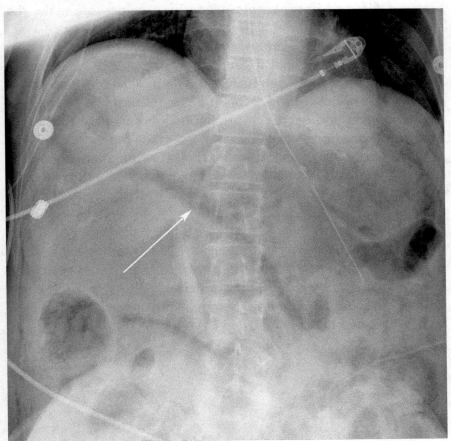

Portal venous gas

The darker tubular structure (arrow) represents gas in the patient's portal vein, the main vein draining blood from the intestines to the liver. Gas continues into the smaller venous branches within the liver, in the patient's upper right abdomen. This patient died shortly afterward from infarcted bowel which had lost its blood supply.

"There is one more thing to do before we put this case to rest," he continued. "Let me go show these to whoever read the chest film this morning. I don't think the miss, or the delay of a few hours in the diagnosis, made any difference. Still, I'm not fond of missing signs of fatal disease. I'd want somebody to point out something like this to me if I missed it."

There was no remaining treatment for the patient once the fatal diagnosis was made. Copies of her x-ray films remain in my teaching file, and in my memory, and have helped me make the same diagnosis in other equally unfortunate individuals since.

Out of internship and new to my specialty field, I was also struck by the distance that so often exists between the patient and the radiologist. Even though there is usually a clear contribution—in this case the discovery and recognition of her terminal diagnosis—the disconnect and degree of separation were palpable. Whether by doing procedures, checking patients' scans during acquisition, asking questions to get a little more clinical information, or directly reviewing results together at times, radiologists do get to interact with patients more than one might think—but there are so many more whom we never directly meet.

Her doctors in the intensive care unit would examine her one more time, discuss her poor prognosis with her family, try to keep her comfortable, and write her last medical chart notes. Perhaps a clergyman read the woman her last rites. I read her last films, which revealed the root of her mortal demise, but never actually laid eyes on her. She died that evening.

SECTION II: DISCOVERIES

T he role of imaging in patient care today cannot be overstated. As mentioned in the introduction, within only a generation or so the field of radiology has bloomed beyond basic x-ray tests to include ultrasound, CT (computed tomography), MRI (magnetic resonance imaging), and new nuclear medicine studies including PET (positron emission tomography). These imaging studies provide roadmaps for doctors to treat all kinds of conditions sooner and more effectively, outlining our organs and diseases like pages from an atlas. Diagnoses help doctors know which medicines to prescribe and give surgeons a much better idea of what they will find in the operating room, making surgery more focused and less exploratory. Even autopsies are performed considerably less often than they used to be, because we usually already know what is wrong with people, and why they die, if they were imaged while still alive.

Medical students get introduced to some imaging studies in classroom courses, but the pictures come to life when students meet and help treat patients in the final years of school. Making sense of the images is often a challenge; it requires explanation, and a great amount of repetition.

For doctors who specialize in radiology after internship, there is a steep learning curve, but a plethora of fascination. I have worked in this field for over a quarter century, and although the interpretation of many cases inevitably becomes routine, it is also true that there is always something new, something different, just

41

like the people being imaged. For myself and every other colleague I have ever asked, interpreting studies is never boring. Mixed among the normal studies and the common abnormalities are the occasional rare diagnoses, or the unusual appearances and atypical presentations that make diagnosis and interventional procedures challenging and rewarding.

I also remain aware that something common on imaging is hardly routine for the patient. Every day that I read CT scans, I diagnose kidney stones being passed. Every evening that I read bone x-rays from the emergency room, there will be fractures. Every weekend that I interpret ultrasound studies, there is usually a first trimester miscarriage. These are commonly occurring conditions, usually with no long-term debilitation for the patient—but I know that most patients will never forget when they had their kidney stone, their fracture, or their miscarriage.

―――――⌘―――――

Residency programs offer incredible learning opportunities under the tutelage of academic professors, along with the hierarchy of fellows and residents, eager to learn together while seeing interesting cases. Regular lectures enhance the education considerably, whether the conferences focus on imaging different conditions, the underlying disease processes, or the physics behind the technology.

While the daytime educational work is more supervised, the regular night call that residents in training must undergo provides opportunities to think independently and make decisions. Residents' overnight cases and interpretations are reviewed with educational feedback provided, but in my era, and at some teaching hospitals still, not until the next morning. Residents generally first learn to make the diagnoses that will keep people alive through the night, for example sending those who need surgery to the operating room; diagnosing infections so that treatment can start; or finding blood clots so that anticoagulation can begin. On the job training is as prevalent, and as useful, in medicine as it can be in other careers.

One of the more rewarding aspects of radiology can be the interaction with and learning from doctors in other specialties.

Dermatologists, who treat our most superficial side, and psychiatrists, who arguably treat the deepest parts of people, order few imaging tests. Just about all other types of doctors order plenty. Radiologists commonly interact with surgeons, emergency physicians, oncologists, pediatricians, obstetricians and gynecologists, internists, and family practitioners. While we aim to help the patients first and serve their primary doctors, we also get to learn a lot in the process.

Perhaps the most important take-home message has been to ever appreciate good health, and to try to do what we can to maintain it. Seeing what I see at work reminds me to be grateful for every day that I am on my side of the x-rays.

PEACE

It was another busy night on call as a resident at the university hospital. I was way behind. The emergency department had ordered so many CT scans that I was beginning to wonder if the ER doctors ordered the scans first and got around to meeting and examining the patients later. In the midst of CT scans on patients who had suffered car wrecks, seizures, or abdominal pain, one emergency doctor also ordered an abdominal ultrasound on a man she suspected had gallstones. At that time of night, there was no tech on call to do the scan—just me. All of the studies were on film then, not yet digital, and each section of the radiology department had its own location, on different floors of the hospital, which meant a lot of back and forth moving around, and a steady stream of pager activity.

I had briefly stopped reading CT scans in order to help an emergency room resident, who had paged me to the ER to look at an x-ray to make sure a patient did not have a fractured neck.

The doctor who had ordered the ultrasound saw me reading the neck x-ray and came over. "You got the message about that ultrasound, right?" she asked.

"I sure did," I acknowledged. "I'll get to it as soon as I can."

"All right, please do," she said.

I intended to, but sicker patients in the same emergency room were taking priority. Reading the films on a patient who had been assaulted, and another with appendicitis, took precedence.

An hour later I got paged to the ER for about the fifteenth time that evening.

"The doctor was wondering when you are going to do that ultrasound," the secretary asked. "She wants to discharge this man, and we could use the room."

"I told her I'll do it as soon as I can. You of all people know what else is going on in that ER tonight. I assure you I'm not watching TV or sleeping."

"I know," she half-apologized, "but the doctor did ask me to call."

"And I thank you for calling, but I've got to get back to work," I replied.

Another half-hour passed, and the CT scanners kept pouring out films. A drunk man had crossed against the light and was hit by a car. A young man had punched his girlfriend and had broken her face below her eye. A middle-aged woman had come in with an obvious bowel obstruction on abdominal films, and the surgeons were waiting for the CT reading to see if they needed to operate. A couple of sick patients who had already been in the hospital needed studies as well, including an old woman with signs of a new stroke, and an old man who had started passing blood from his rectum.

Amidst all of this, my pager went off again, summoned by the emergency room. It was the same doctor who had ordered the abdominal ultrasound two hours previously.

"I'm just checking on that ultrasound," she said, with a little more firmness in her voice.

"I take it you're not working on the trauma or surgical side of your department tonight, or you would already know the answer to your question. I really am going as fast as I can, and trying to take care of the sickest people first."

"I respect that," she began, "but we do have issues of turnaround time that we like to stick to."

"Unfortunately, the hospital currently does not pay for ultrasound techs to take call, as you know. I'm all you've got. Your secretary said you're going to discharge him. Does he really have to be done tonight? We'd be happy to scan him as an outpatient tomorrow daytime, when there are more people here besides me."

"We prefer to get a diagnosis before we send people out the door," she explained.

"I'll tell you what," I said. "If you promise not to call me about it again, and if you explain to your colleagues why they might have

45

a brief delay in some of their CT readings, send him down in ten minutes and I'll do it."

I was in the hallway outside the ultrasound scanning room twelve minutes later. The patient was nowhere to be found. I waited five minutes, then called the ER. I got the same secretary who had been nice to me earlier.

"This is your chance for that man's ultrasound," I said.

"Transport is wheeling him out right now," she insisted.

A few minutes later, a young woman wearing dark blue scrubs walked off the elevator while pushing a wheelchair. In the chair sat a fat man, his knees pointed off to the sides. His belly made a round mound below his light blue cotton gown, raising the hemline so high that it barely covered his genital area. Thick, fleshy thighs spread out over the entire seat of the wheelchair.

I had met this young transporter on a number of other nights. She was petite, quiet and patient, with a pleasantness that somehow survived all of the ravages and demands of her working environment. Tonight, pushing that large man in the wheelchair, she also proved that she had more upper body strength than I would have ever imagined.

"Thanks," I said to her.

"Thank you," she said, smiling back, then left him with me.

I introduced myself to the man, who was, fortunately, able to get up out of the wheelchair and lie down on the stretcher unassisted.

"If I'd known I would have been here this long already, I might have thought of staying home, only if that pain hadn't been so bad," he shrugged. "You've got a busy hospital going here."

"You better believe it," I said. "Let's take a look at your belly while we've finally got a chance. Where are you hurting the most?"

"I'm not hurting now," he explained, "but I was at home a few hours ago after supper, and it hurt right over here," he pointed toward his upper right abdomen.

I began scanning his abdomen. Given his size, it was not easy. In the midst of trying to see what I could, my pager suddenly went off twice in rapid succession, both times to the ER. They meant business.

"Excuse me," I apologized. "I need to call the emergency room."

"That's quite all right," he said, resting comfortably on the stretcher in the dark room. "From all the hollering in there, I know they've got people in worse shape than me."

I dialed the number on my pager and was connected to the same doctor who had ordered this man's abdominal ultrasound. "We need you for a STAT ultrasound in the ER," she said. "We just got a call that an ambulance is arriving in about one minute with someone who may be having a ruptured aortic aneurysm."

"I can do that, but you know I'm in the middle of scanning the man you were waiting for me to bring down for so long."

"He can wait," she urged. "We need you here more."

"OK, send a transporter to get him back to the ER. I'm on my way." I apologized to the man, had him climb down off the table into the wheelchair, and pushed him into the long, empty hospital basement corridor, where I left him sitting alone and unattended, something I cannot imagine doing today. I then pushed the ultrasound machine, even larger and more cumbersome than he was in the wheelchair, onto the elevator and went straight to the ER.

I never finished the study on the man I had left in the hallway. He was discharged after all, with an order to schedule his ultrasound as an outpatient, just as I had suggested before.

By the time I arrived in the emergency department, a group of paramedics was hoisting a backboard onto a stretcher. On the board lay a motionless, elderly, emaciated man. A throng of residents and medical students prepared to pounce into his resuscitation, like a frenzy in green hospital scrubs.

The doctor who had paged me to do the ultrasound was at a desk outside the room, speaking on the telephone. A different emergency physician, a tall man in regular pants, a buttoned shirt, and a long white coat, was in charge, or as in charge as anyone could try to be, given the mystery and gravity of the unknown patient's condition, and the chaos that resulted in the crowded room. Paramedics were calling out what medicines they had already administered and what little they knew about the pale, unresponsive man. Nurses were hooking up more oxygen and intravenous fluids, while someone was shouting out details of the man's abnormal heart rhythm. The resident in charge of resuscitation codes that night was warming up the defibrillator paddles.

"Do you still want me to check for a triple-A?" I called to the head doctor, referring to an abdominal aortic aneurysm.

"Go ahead since you're here," he motioned, then turned to the sea of green-clad residents. "Step back folks and make some room!"

Resuscitation efforts continued. Amidst cries of no detectable pulse or blood pressure, I tried to scan the man's abdomen while other residents began giving chest compressions. The pictures I tried to take during the commotion were certainly not my finest. Of all the resuscitation codes I had been involved in during medical school and internship, there had never been a radiologist there. My presence was a rarity, a consequence of unusual timing and coincidence.

As difficult as it was to scan a man undergoing CPR, I could tell them that he had no fluid in his abdomen and that his aorta was not dilated. Whatever he was dying of, it was not a ruptured abdominal aortic aneurysm. I moved out of the way and headed to the periphery of the crowd, watching in silence.

"Hold compression and let's get another tracing," the doctor in charge ordered. The old man's heart did show an electrical rhythm with a normal rate on the monitor.

"He's got a rhythm," someone called out.

"I can't feel a pulse," said a resident with his fingers on the man's neck.

"I don't hear one either," said another resident, listening to the man's chest with a stethoscope.

"How much epinephrine has he gotten?" someone asked.

"He needs an amp of bicarb by now," the head doctor ordered. "Resume compression!"

A resident continued compressing the old man's chest, sometimes making cracking noises when pushing on his sternum, while someone else squeezed the ventilation bag attached to the patient's face mask.

The chief resident climbed above the patient. Her long hair

was pulled back behind her neck, and she held a defibrillator paddle in each hand. "We're not getting anywhere," she said, "and I'm shocking him."

"He has a rhythm, Christine," the tall emergency doctor in charge scolded. "That's not the thing to do."

"Well I don't care!" she snapped, frustrated at not being able to use the tools she held, while the old man lay dying despite the other resuscitation efforts.

"Check your ACLS manual," he yelled.

"I did, and I'm trying to save him," she yelled back.

"You're not following the algorithm," he berated. "I *wrote* the chapter, and he does not need defibrillation with that rhythm. What he needs is for his heart to start contracting, soon."

"All clear!" she yelled as the residents stopped CPR and everyone stood back. She put the paddles on the man's chest and delivered the electrical shock, then removed her paddles.

A weak EKG rhythm showed on the monitor, not particularly different than before the jolt, and not any more effective.

"I still can't hear a heartbeat," said the resident with the stethoscope on the man's chest.

"No pulse either," said the resident feeling the old man's neck.

Someone started resuming chest compressions when the head doctor called out: "Is radiology still here?"

"Yes," I answered, stepping forward at the surprise summons.

"Can you use this ultrasound here to scan his heart?" he asked. The idea had not occurred to me before his request.

"Sure," I said. I did not know how to do a thorough echocardiogram to study heart valves and wall muscles, but I could at least find the man's heart to watch it beat. The residents stopped their compressions. Quickly I squirted gel on his chest with one hand and grabbed the scanning transducer with the other, placing it in the gel on his chest between two ribs.

I pointed to a doughnut-shaped structure on the screen while the crowd watched. His heart quivered once, its last time, then stopped, perfectly still.

"This is his left ventricle in cross-section," I explained, "and it's not moving."

The room had suddenly gone quiet, as all of us looked at the undeniable visual evidence that this man was dying before us. All of the doctors and nurses in the resuscitation code knew the man was likely not going to make it, but seeing his motionless heart on the ultrasound somehow convinced everyone even more completely than the heart monitor and failing vital signs.

"He's flat-lining now," someone yelled.

"*Now* you can shock," the tall doctor in charge said to the chief resident, "*one* more time." I jumped back with the rest of them.

The doctor who had called me to do the ultrasound was standing in the doorway of the bay. She could tell the resuscitation was failing.

"Do we know anything about this guy yet?" the tall male doctor asked the crowd.

"I just spoke with a family member," she answered from the doorway. "He's been getting treatments for cancer for some time now, and was not expected to live much longer."

"Have they ever heard of hospice?" the tall doctor grumbled, shaking his head.

They stopped the code shortly afterward. The resuscitation room got quiet again. The horde of students and residents milled around in the hallway for a moment, and then dispersed. With other patients to treat, we all went back to our various duties for the rest of the dark hours.

Morning finally came. While the deceased man's family dealt with the aftermath of his turbulent passing, morning rounds and shift changes came for the overnight staff. We all checked in with the new, rested crews relieving us. While they geared up for another day and night ahead, those of us ending our shifts sought to find solace from the chaos of the night before. I began by going home to sleep.

BLOCKED

"**H**ave you ever had this test before?" I asked the young woman sitting between the stirrups mounted on the examination table at the city hospital. She sheepishly shook her head no. She was shy, or perhaps just nervous. She was twenty-nine according to the birth date on her paperwork, and some of those twenty-nine years must have been rough. Her hair was brown, flat, nondescript. Her skin was pale, and her face already revealed a few subtle lines which left her looking slightly aged, like someone who had had to work harder, or worry more, than some of her peers.

She had never been pregnant, despite being in a relationship with a boyfriend for several years. Her use of contraception had gone from routine, to sporadic, to infrequent. If she was not actively trying to have a child at that time, she was obviously open to the possibility. Because she had still never been pregnant, she was beginning to wonder if she could conceive at all.

She had made an appointment with a gynecologist at the public clinic. Regardless of the contraceptive issues they might need to discuss, the history was concerning enough that the clinic physician wanted to make sure that the young woman would someday be able to conceive. She ordered an x-ray study called a hysterosalpingogram, or HSG.

"It looks like your urine pregnancy test was negative this morning. Are your menstrual cycles regular every month?" I asked the woman, while a female x-ray tech wrote down the information the patient revealed.

"Yes," she said.

"And your last one started when?"

"Seven days ago."

"OK. Have you ever had any pelvic surgery?" I asked.

"No."

"Ever been told that you have a condition called endometriosis?" I inquired.

"No," she shook her head.

"And have you ever had any pelvic infection?"

"Yes, once," she admitted.

"A significant one? Were you admitted to the hospital?"

"Yeah, for several days. They gave me antibiotics in my arm. That was the one time, about five years ago."

"I don't know what your doctor may have told you about this test," I began. "It starts out sort of like a Pap smear; we place a speculum below."

She nodded without speaking a word.

"But instead of doing a Pap smear," I continued, "we place a small, sterile catheter in the cervix. Through that I'll gently inject a little contrast fluid that shows up on the x-ray. That will let us see the inside of your uterus, and if your Fallopian tubes are open."

She nodded, quietly, slightly apprehensive.

"It only takes a few minutes. Most women feel just a little cramping while the fluid is being injected, but it goes away as soon as we're done. You may also have a little spotting over the next day or so, on account of the catheter being placed briefly."

"OK," she said, looking resigned to getting the study completed.

The x-ray tech assisting me had the young woman lie back and place her feet in the stirrups at the table's edge. I lubricated the speculum with sterile gel, placed it below, and swabbed antiseptic onto her cervix. The x-ray tech adjusted the lamp over my shoulder, shining light onto the woman's cervix, and the catheter was easily placed.

"You may feel some cramping while I start the fluid injection," I warned. The patient closed her eyes just slightly as the injection began, while the x-ray tech comforted her by rubbing the woman's hand, advising slow, deep breaths.

We watched the x-ray monitor screen. Her uterus filled normally. The contrast then readily flowed into her right Fallopian tube, and at first appeared to swirl freely into the pelvis beyond the normally thin tube segment attached to the uterus, as a healthy tube should. However, no contrast fluid entered the tube on the other side.

"I do feel cramping," she said, slightly uncomfortable.

"It'll be just a couple of minutes at most," I said. "I need to see the left side fill. If you can bear it, I need to increase the pressure a little." I slightly increased the pressure on the syringe, and she put one hand on her forehead. Contrast kept filling the right tube, and the appearance of the tube was changing as it filled with the additional fluid. The right tube was normal in caliber near the uterus, then abnormally distended farther away from the uterus, an elongated balloon shape that blindly tapered to a point—a shape I had never seen before. The left tube never filled and remained invisible.

"It won't be much longer," the x-ray tech assured her.

"We're almost done," I agreed. A final push on the syringe only increased the pressure of her cramping, and did not propel contrast any farther out the tubes. I took out the catheter and speculum.

"All done," I said.

She sighed, relieved. "It wasn't as bad as I thought it was going to be. How does it look?"

"I'm not sure," I began, truthfully. "Your left tube does look blocked. At first I thought the right one is open, but I want to show these films to a colleague here and get another opinion."

She looked at me quizzically, but seemed hesitant to ask anything.

"Remember," I told her, "you only need one tube to be open in order to get pregnant. If just one Fallopian tube is open, you can usually still get pregnant, but only every other month on average, depending on which ovary is releasing an egg any given month."

She had gotten her feet out of the stirrups and sat up on the x-ray table, looking eager to get dressed and go.

"I'll get this report to your doctor soon," I said, and left the exam room.

When the films had printed, I reviewed them with my radiology professor. "I've got an HSG to show you. I've only done a few so far, and the others were normal. I don't think this one is going to be."

"How did it go?"

"OK, technically. I was able to do the study. But it's abnormal. The left tube is definitely blocked. It didn't fill at all. And the more I look at these films, maybe the other side doesn't look right, either."

We looked at the pictures together while I explained. "At first I thought the right tube was going to be fine. It filled, and it looked like it was open, with contrast spilling out into the pelvis. Only it didn't freely float away; it stayed trapped in one pocket here," I pointed.

"Yes, I see that. And it never went beyond this collection."

"No. Now that we've got the films to review, no, now I don't think it did."

"And the contrast is in the shape of a dilated tube," he said. "She's got a hydrosalpinx."

"So you think this whole thing is just a big, dilated Fallopian tube? All of it?"

"Yes, I do," he said. "They can get this large, and that's exactly the shape you'd expect."

Even if her Fallopian tube had been open—and hers was not—the tube likely would not have worked properly. An egg would have trouble being propelled through an abnormally dilated tube, unlikely to make it from the ovary to her uterus. Her tube was not only dilated, but closed off on its outer aspect, near the ovary. An egg would not be able to enter that Fallopian tube in the first place.

"And her other tube is blocked as well," he said. "So she's sterile."

There it was: the explanation, the result, the outcome. She had the history of pelvic inflammatory disease in her past from a prior bacterial infection, the most common sexually transmitted bacteria being gonorrhea and chlamydia. One unfortunate exposure had left lingering, lifelong consequences. The infection caused scars she was not even aware of, scar tissue that distorted her reproductive tract, making it nonfunctional. Yet this scarring not only affected her body; it interrupted her biological input to the next generation and beyond. Without fertility treatments quite advanced for that time, which she could probably not afford, this woman would likely never conceive a child of her own.

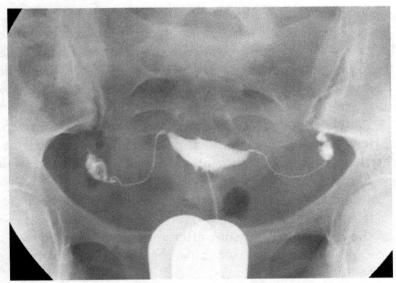

Normal Fallopian tubes on a hysterosalpingogram
The central white density is contrast within the uterus. The thin white curved lines extending to each side of the pelvis represent contrast within normal Fallopian tubes

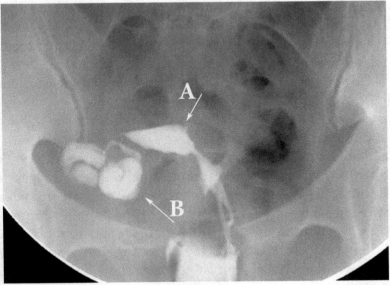

The patient's left Fallopian tube (A) does not fill with the bright contrast fluid injected. This tube is blocked from scar tissue formation. The patient's right Fallopian tube (B) fills but is abnormally dilated, called a hydrosalpinx, and is also closed at its outer end.

"What did you tell her?" the professor asked.

"I told her that the left side was blocked, and I'd have to look at the case with you before we issue the final report. But I didn't say there was definitely a problem on the right, as it looks like now. Only when I got the films printed, and reviewed them here with you, do I see the full extent."

I thought about her receiving that unexpected and unwelcome news from one of the clinic doctors. This woman would not be prepared to hear that result, after our limited and incomplete review of her images.

"She already left. I better call her and let her know the full story."

I telephoned her later that day. "I did review your case with one of the radiology professors, after you left. He agreed that the left side was blocked, but it looks like there's also a problem on the right side, too."

She just listened. I kept talking.

"After looking at your pictures more, it looks as if your right tube is abnormally dilated, and also closed at its outer end, toward the ovary." I left it at there for a moment. She remained silent on the other end of the line. "So although most of it filled, that tube's not really open." She did not say anything.

"Do you have any questions?" I asked. She did not, at least at the immediate moment.

"Do you have an appointment in the clinic to see your doctor again?"

"They told me to schedule one after this test," she said softly.

"Be sure to do that, so they can go over these results with you more," I advised. Quietly she thanked me for calling.

Ten days later I tried to borrow the woman's images from the hospital film library, to show them at a teaching conference. "They're checked out to the gynecology clinic," the file room clerk told me. "They often do that for patients' appointments—they'll send them back eventually, but if you need them sooner and want to run down there, they might let you have them if they don't need them anymore."

I went to the clinic and was led to a nurse's office. She looked up from her desk, where she was writing notes in patients' charts. I introduced myself and explained what I was looking for.

"Her films? Yes, I've got them right here," she said, motioning me to a chair across from her. She grabbed the film folder from a stack propped against the side of her desk. "We saw her back a few days ago. As you can imagine, she's just devastated about this."

"She seemed kind of passive when I spoke to her, almost receptive," I replied.

"She may be like that, but this news hit her pretty hard," the nurse revealed.

"I don't guess there's any surgery that could be done to open these up?" I questioned.

"Not at this point, nothing with any good success rate," she said.

"And in vitro is probably way too expensive?" I asked, knowing that the woman received her care at the public hospital clinic.

"She's a waitress with no health insurance," she said. "Unless her circumstances change unexpectedly in the future, it's simply not an option for her."

I have no idea if she ever acquired the means to pay, or if she is still paying emotionally. Clearly there is so much more to people's lives than the children they produce, but without a small miracle, a big component of the life she may have dreamed about will likely never come to fruition.

ALIEN

Mike spoke to his patient on the CT scanner through the control room microphone. "Hold still, sir. *¡No se mueve, señor!*" Evidently unsuccessful with his command, Mike shook his head in exasperation, then saw me enter the room. "You speak Spanish, don't you?" he asked.

"*Sí,*" I replied.

"This guy just won't hold still. I don't know if it's from his illness, or if he just doesn't understand me," Mike said in frustration.

"What's he having done?" I asked.

"Just a head CT, for a new onset of seizures. Do you think you could talk to him?"

"Sure, I'll try."

I went in and met the middle-aged Mexican man. Not currently convulsing, he appeared mildly dazed and lethargic in his post seizure state. Conversing in Spanish, I introduced myself and asked him how he was feeling.

"I'm all right," he said.

"Do you know where you are, sir?" I asked.

"The hospital."

"And do you understand why you are here?" I asked.

"My family called the ambulance."

"Why?"

"They said I was having convulsions."

"Have you ever had this before?"

"No, never," he said.

Briefly I thought of the possible reasons that a person his age might develop seizures for the first time. Epilepsy might, or might not, be the culprit. He could have a brain tumor, an electrolyte disturbance from kidney damage, a stroke, bleeding from high blood pressure, even a ruptured brain aneurysm. Other possibilities included side effects from alcohol or drug abuse, although he did not look like a hardcore drug user. It could even be from a bad reaction to medication. The CT scan was an important first step in figuring out the cause.

"Sir, this young man needs to take some pictures of your head, and it's important that you hold still. It's quick. Do you think you can try not to move for about one minute when he tells you?"

"*Sí doctor.*"

I turned back to Mike, the CT tech. "Give it a try, he'll do his best."

Looking through the glass separating our two rooms, Mike and I could see that the patient was resting quietly. Mike was able to complete the study within a few minutes. I stayed to watch and began reviewing the images as they came up on the computer screen.

This was no normal brain.

"What the heck is that?" Mike asked me. "That's not like any brain tumor I've ever seen."

"No, it's definitely not. In fact, it may not be a tumor at all. Give me a minute to look at this." It only took a few moments to rule out a few important conditions: There was no sign of bleeding, or stroke, and I did not think he had an actual tumor. The normal regions containing cerebrospinal fluid were not dilated. His brain also showed no sign of atrophy commonly seen in alcoholics. There was, however, a large, abnormal cystic cavity containing fluid, with a small amount of solid debris near the periphery, and several small calcifications scattered elsewhere throughout his brain tissue.

"They ordered it without initially, but with contrast at your discretion," Mike explained. "Should I inject him? His IV is ready to go."

"Yeah, go ahead. He may need an MRI anyway, but while he's on the table and cooperative, give him some contrast and let's see how this thing enhances."

I went back into the scanner room with the scanner and continued speaking Spanish to the man, still lying on the table.

"Sir, you did very well."

"*Gracias, doctor.*"

"There is something I want to get a better look at," I explained. "We are now going to give you an injection in your IV, while we take a few more pictures, so that we can see more."

"*Sí doctor, está bien.*"

"Do you have any allergies to any medicines that you know of?"

"*No.*"

"Very well, this will be just like before, only he will take the pictures while he is injecting a little fluid through your IV. You may feel warm during the injection, and your mouth may taste like metal for a moment, but usually that's all. This part is important to see things a little better."

"*Sí doctor.*"

The man did fine with the injection, and again held reasonably still. When the pictures began to appear on the computer screen, we could see that there was above average blood flow enhancing the wall of the large cyst, indicating an active process, rather than something old that had been there for years. In addition, one small spot of solid tissue at the cyst wall lit up brightly.

"I want to see this area on the pre-contrast study again," I said. "Can we zoom up on these slices?"

Mike gave me the images to study while he got the patient off the CT scanner table and helped him back onto his stretcher. Mike looked at me through the glass window, befuddled with his limited Spanish while trying to understand the patient, while still curious to understand the nature of the man's illness just shown on the scan. Asking only with his eyes, he summoned me back into the room with the patient.

Having seen this man's disease several times in other Latino patients, I made the probable diagnosis in only a few minutes. Something small had invaded the sanctity of his brain tissue by way of his bloodstream, and had taken up residence there. An inflammatory reaction had formed a walled-off pocket of fluid, which compressed the adjacent brain tissue.

"He's asking something," Mike said as I re-entered the room.

"*Sí, señor,*" I asked the gentleman, who was alert enough to initiate conversation, and at this point understandably inquisitive.

"*Doctor, ¿qué ve en el estudio?*" the man asked, wanting to know what we had found, revealing just a hint of anxiety.

I hesitated. He noticed. I explained that we had found an abnormality.

He looked at me quizzically. "*¿Es cáncer?*"

"*No señor, no es tumor. Creo que es una infección.*"

"*¿Infección? Como un virus?*"

"*No señor, no es virus.*"

He studied me with puzzled anticipation, awaiting my explanation:

"*Parece como un parásito.*"

"*¡Un parásito!*" he exclaimed, despite his weakness. "*En el cerebro?*" he sighed, staring at the ceiling in combined horror and exhaustion. "*O Dios, no.*"

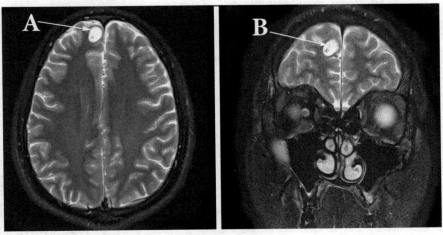

Cysticercosis
Brain MRI axial (A) and coronal (B) images in a patient
with cysticercosis (tapeworm larvae infection).
—Images courtesy of Oluwatoyin Idowu, MD

I tried to minimize the impact, continuing to explain in Spanish. "It's a small parasite, almost microscopic. Not like in the intestine. And it can be treated."

"*¿Sí? Gracias a Dios. Gracias, doctor.*" Having processed all the unwelcome information he could in the fatigue of his post-convulsive state, he closed his eyes and tried to rest, temporarily putting aside thoughts of the small creatures affecting his mind by literally invading its tissue.

Later, after the patient was back in the emergency room before formal admission to the hospital, Mike and I again reviewed the images on our computer screen.

"I've seen these small calcifications a number of times before, almost always in Hispanic patients," he said. "But never anything like that big cyst there, with that little spot inside that you pointed out."

"Fortunately, no. But that's what an acute infection can look like. The small calcifications are from old infections that have scarred down, where the larvae have died. That one with the cyst and peripheral blood flow is likely still alive. *Cysticercosis*, the tapeworm larva.

'Man, don't drink the water."

"Actually, it's usually from eating pork that's not adequately cooked—which is one more reason I'll be dining veggie tonight. I read once that this is the number one diagnosis for people in Mexico who develop a new onset of seizures."

"So those tiny worms lodge in the brain, and cause a big infection like that? Wow."

"Nasty, huh? The fluid in the cyst is part of the body's immune reaction to the larvae. A lot of the complications, like his seizures, are probably caused by the mass effect from the big cyst pushing on the brain tissue."

"But they can cure it?"

"They can treat it. It takes a long time, and it's not always a hundred percent successful, but let's hope it is in him."

CONFESSION

Toward the end of my training, a young woman wearing a white coat came to see me in the hospital reading room. She was holding a small stack of MRI films in her arms. Her patient had just had the study done and left the department.

"Hi, I'm one of the residents on the transplant service," she began. "I was hoping you could look at these films with me."

"Looks like they're hot off the press," I teased. "What's the story?"

"He's a Catholic priest in his mid-sixties with cirrhosis, which we think may be due to hemochromatosis." She was referring to an inherited disorder that causes excess iron storage in the liver. The iron overload damages the liver cells and can cause cirrhosis by middle age.

"He had negative blood tests for hepatitis B and C," she continued, "and is only a social drinker. We ordered the MRI to see how bad his liver looks, and as part of his transplant evaluation. He shouldn't need a transplant right away, but he might be headed in that direction, so we've got his work-up underway."

We hung the films up on the fluorescent-lit view boxes. The sheets of film contained over 200 small pictures to review, but it did not take much time for me to doubt the disease that she and the transplant team had considered.

"How did the diagnosis of hemochromatosis get made?" I asked. "Was it confirmed on a liver biopsy?"

She thought to herself briefly, then replied, "No, he has not had a liver biopsy recently, and his iron levels are pending. We don't know yet that his iron is elevated, but it's high in our differential, because there is some vague family history of liver disease, and the more common causes have been ruled out."

"He doesn't have hemochromatosis. Look at these images here. If he had excess iron stored in his liver, the liver would look a lot darker on these pictures. Here the tissue is fine, at least in terms of iron level."

"That's very interesting," she said. "I think that maybe we were considering that diagnosis because we don't have another explanation yet. How bad does the cirrhosis look?"

I studied the rest of the images of his liver. Cirrhosis was not his only trouble.

"He's got a problem," I said pointing to the most important pictures on the films. "The cirrhosis is fairly pronounced, but look at these slices here. He's got small tumors in his liver, four of them. From the blood flow pattern, they're probably malignant."

"Do you mean metastases?" she asked. "He's got no known history of cancer."

"They don't have to be metastases. It could be multifocal primary liver cancer."

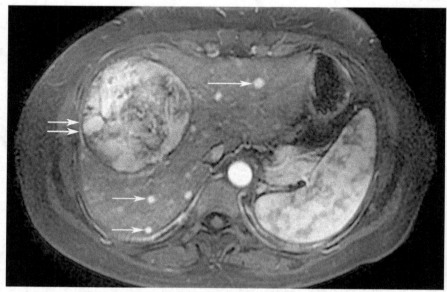

Liver cancers (multifocal hepatocellular carcinoma)
In another patient with cirrhosis, the large mass (double arrow) is a liver cancer. The small white lesions (single arrows) are additional cancers also originating in the liver.

Liver cells that have been damaged for years are more likely to become cancerous. Because a liver with cirrhosis is damaged throughout, there is fairly equal potential for damaged cells to deteriorate to cancer at any given site within the organ. Therefore, liver cancer in a patient with cirrhosis might develop in only one spot, or it may arise in several areas fairly simultaneously.

We continued looking at the films together. In addition to the cirrhosis, he had other complications, including an enlarged spleen, dilated veins, and mild fluid within his abdomen. All are abnormalities that can occur with cirrhosis of almost any cause.

However, I saw another abnormality that shed light on the real reason this man had cirrhosis of the liver.

"You said that he has never had cancer before, right? That would include prostate cancer?"

"That's right," she confirmed. "We screened him for prostate cancer as part of his workup. His PSA was normal."

"So I assume he's not taking any kind of testosterone-blocking medicine?"

"No," she denied.

I pointed to the front of his chest. "Look here. This is a lot more breast tissue than a man should have, even at his age. This man has gynecomastia," I said, using the medical term for prominent breast tissue within a man.

"What does that have to do with his liver?" she asked.

"You tell me. If this man were being treated for prostate cancer with testosterone-blocking drugs, that would be one explanation for his gynecomastia. Since that's not the case, what's another explanation?"

She thought for a moment. "I suppose anything that would lower his testosterone level."

"Right. Now, given that the last operatic castrato died a long time ago, we'll assume this man has testicles. In fact, we can see them right here," I pointed, "but barely, because his are small."

"So they're atrophied. Which could explain the prominent breast tissue," she nodded.

"Exactly. Okay, so what's the missing link here? Since it doesn't look like excessive iron causing his liver damage, what is the most likely explanation that this man would have testicular atrophy and cirrhosis?" I asked.

She paused for another moment. "Alcohol?" she proposed, hesitating in her reply, but displaying a mild sparkle of revelation in her eye.

"Bingo," I replied. "I suppose we can't say that for sure, but it's by far the most likely cause, and the one thing that ties all of this together neatly."

"Wow," she said. "On more than one occasion we've asked him about his level of drinking. He admits to maybe a couple of drinks a day, but has never acknowledged more than that."

"That could be a red flag right there. Somebody with cirrhosis shouldn't drink at all, certainly not every day."

"No, of course not," she replied. "Now that I think about it, he didn't elaborate much on his actual intake, but we gathered that it's less now that he's been diagnosed with liver disease. He never indicated any problem."

"You've heard the joke about how to tell when an alcoholic is lying to you?" I asked.

"Yeah, I know," she said, "when his lips are moving..." She paused, looking more serious. "The rest of the transplant team is going to be really interested to hear this. It's a shame we didn't figure this out sooner."

"It might not have mattered, if he wasn't ready to do anything about it. And if it's this hard to get an accurate alcohol intake from a priest, it shows how challenging it can be sometimes to get a reliable history."

"This is going to make it a lot harder for him to get a transplant," she said from concern.

"Yeah, I imagine so. How long do you all require that an alcoholic quit drinking before getting on the list as a liver transplant candidate? Six months, right?"

"At least six months," she responded.

When the transplant doctors confronted the priest, he was reluctant to acknowledge the extent of his drinking, at least initially. Eventually, however, he admitted that he had significantly underestimated the quantity of alcohol he regularly consumed.

His surgeons outlined his situation clearly: they could not selectively cut out the tumors in his diseased liver. The man's best chance for survival would be a liver transplant—provided he could stop drinking long enough to be considered for an organ donation, and provided that his liver cancer did not spread to other parts of his body in the meantime. Yet the cirrhosis, and the tumors growing within his damaged liver, turned out to be more determined than his resolve to quit drinking.

Ultimate Denial

A woman in her mid-thirties felt a breast lump a few months after she stopped breastfeeding her one-year-old child, the youngest of her several children. Her doctor ordered a mammogram. When Shelby, the technologist, brought me the films, the concern on her face was evident. Together we looked at the mammogram and quickly knew that trouble lay ahead, but we did not realize how much trouble.

"Her mammogram could have come right out of a radiology textbook," I said, and Shelby agreed. The films showed a classically suspicious cluster of small calcifications. There was almost no question that she had breast cancer.

We walked down the hall together to the patient, who was still waiting in the examination room. I shook her hand while introducing myself and hung her films on a view box on the wall.

"You do have an abnormality, right where you feel that lump, in this spot here," I pointed out. "The appearance is suspicious, and I'm going to recommend that you have a biopsy."

She remained attentive and calm. Small tears ran from the corner of each eye. She wiped them away with a finger. "My doctor thought it might just be a cyst."

"I know." Before the study, her doctor would have probably been right statistically, but all of that changed with the mammogram. "Unfortunately, that's not how it looks."

"I understand." She looked down for a moment, wiping another tear.

After asking a few more questions, the young woman thanked us and left. I telephoned the surgeon who had ordered the mammogram when he had seen the woman in the clinic. He arranged for her to have a breast biopsy. Everything seemed in order.

Several weeks later, I saw the same surgeon in the hospital. "Hey," I asked him, "how did things turn out with the young mother with the breast lump and the abnormal mammogram?"

He ran his dark brown hand across his smooth scalp and sighed. "You won't believe it. We did her biopsy right in the clinic, since we could feel the lump, and it came back ductal carcinoma *in situ*. The pathologist said it was clearly cancerous, but she couldn't see any invasion of the surrounding tissue. Yet after the biopsy results came back, the patient is refusing to have the surgery to remove it. I'm not sure that she believes she has cancer. I think she freaked out from the news, and we can't get her back into the office."

My eyes widened. If the woman waited too long before having the cancer removed, it could become invasive. Of the different types of breast cancer, hers was the easiest to cure. A delay in treatment could squander the opportunity that the early diagnosis provided.

"You can't be serious. How could anybody ignore a positive biopsy result, particularly someone so young, and with children no less?"

"I know," he said, shaking his head again. "Our nurse has tried to get her to schedule the lumpectomy. The patient will not return our calls."

His revelation was unbelievable to me. "Does she have any psychiatric history?"

"Not that we know of," he sighed. "As far as we can tell, she's competent to make this decision, even if it seems crazy to us."

I could not stop thinking about this young woman and her family, whom I had never met. Her young children could lose their mother, by her unwillingness to acknowledge her illness and have it treated. She had the right to make her own decision, but every fiber in me said her decision was simply wrong. Out of fear or misinformation, she was risking her very survival, with devastating potential consequences for her family. She could prevent that outcome.

I paged the surgeon several days later. "I apologize if I might be overstepping my role as a radiologist."

"Not at all," he said.

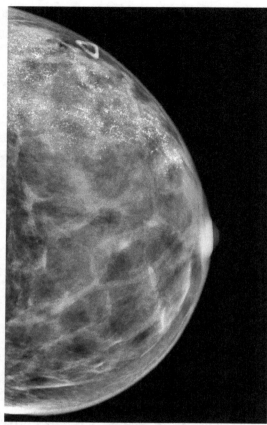

Breast cancer
Mammogram with a malignant cluster of small white calcifications on the upper aspect of the image.

"I just wouldn't feel right if I didn't try to contact her myself. My interaction with her on the day of her mammogram was obviously brief, but it seemed productive, and normal. We communicated well enough for her to get the biopsy at least. Would you object to my calling her, to discuss her treatment further?"

"Please, feel free. Anything that would bring her in for surgery would be great," he encouraged.

Later that day I dialed her number. When she answered the telephone, I took a deep breath, reminding myself to stay reserved. I wanted her to take this seriously, but not to get overly scared into inaction. She might fear the pain, the cosmetic result, or the risks of the operation. She needed to be concerned enough to undergo the surgery, but not too afraid to return to the hospital.

On the contrary, she sounded almost chipper. "I remember you, doctor," she exclaimed. "But I feel fine now. The lump is gone, and everything is okay."

I could not believe my ears. I tried to stay cool and non-confrontational, but I was amazed at her statement.

"I understand that you had your biopsy last month. They did tell you the results, didn't they?"

"Yes, but I am fine now. I'm telling you, it's gone. I can't feel a thing."

"But it's not all gone," I countered. "They didn't take it all out, only a little piece of it with the biopsy. The cancer is still there."

"No, I understand what you're saying, but I really don't think so," she said. Her voice sounded rational, but her statements were far from it.

"I don't mean to contradict you," I continued, "but I have to. It must be difficult to hear news like yours, but your biopsy showed breast cancer. If you have it removed now, you have a good chance of doing just fine. The longer you wait, the greater the chance that it could spread."

"You've all been very nice, and I appreciate your concern," she said, "but I'm doing well now." The level of exchanged information progressed little further from this point. The more I tried to explain that she still had a cancer in her breast, the more emphatically she stated that she no longer had a problem. She thanked me for calling, but she did not budge in her conviction. I gave her my telephone number at work and encouraged her to call the surgeon, or me, if she had any questions.

After the call ended, I envisioned other patients I had known with breast cancer diagnosed later than hers. Many had ended up with metastases and suffered from the pain and debilitation of their disease, not to mention the side effects of radiation and chemotherapy. Some of course did not survive. Would this woman end up like one of those patients, all because she insisted on blowing her opportunity for early treatment and potential cure?

The surgeon was obviously disappointed when I told him of my telephone interaction with the patient. "But," he said, "after talking with her myself, unfortunately I'm not surprised."

With my conscience continuing to haunt me for several weeks afterward, I tried to communicate with her one more time, if for no other reason than to convince myself that I had done everything I knew to do. If the telephone conversation was not fruitful, then perhaps a written letter might be more productive. She could read it and reread it on her own time. Maybe the weight of her diagnosis, and the severity of the consequences by refusing treatment, could sink in eventually. The surgeon had already written a letter but welcomed my trying once more. I sent a letter that was informative but simple to understand, including telephone numbers for the surgeon and myself. She had all of the information I knew to provide her. The surgeon and I would wait for her to make an appointment at the clinic, or to contact one of us.

We waited.

And still we waited.

Four years later, she came into the emergency room, complaining of a painful mass in her breast. The tumor had grown into the skin and started bleeding. The emergency doctors immediately suspected an aggressive breast cancer. They did not imagine, until pouring through her records from four years prior, that she had been diagnosed with cancer back then, but declined all treatment. She had not seen a doctor since that time.

She saw plenty of doctors in the following days, but there was little that any could do. A CT scan revealed metastatic tumors throughout her liver, lungs, and bones. It was far too late to save her with radiation and chemotherapy treatments.

Palliative care was eventually arranged to keep her comfortable, and it was only a matter of months before she succumbed to her disease. I was no longer involved in the case at that point and did not meet her husband or children. A colleague treating her told me that, like many families having to process and cope with the loss of a loved one from terminal illness, her family said they had to accept this as her fate, the decision having been in God's hands.

What the patient's family may not know is that four years previously, the hands of fate may have been her own.

BRAIN DEATH

It started as a routine weekend day shift at the hospital. I was reading studies for the patients already admitted, as well as those coming into the emergency department, when the phone rang midafternoon. Jessie, the nuclear medicine technologist, spoke slowly and clearly on the telephone, his matter-of-fact tone only slightly colored by the ominous nature of the information he conveyed. "Doc, I'll need you to come over in a minute. The ICU has ordered a brain scan on a kid who was in a rollover accident a couple days ago. Apparently he ain't doing too good."

My own heartbeat began to accelerate. Rarely does so much depend upon the interpretation of a single study. Even more rarely, I thought to myself, is there so strong a need to be essentially one hundred percent certain of the interpretation. His doctors in the intensive care unit needed to know if his brain had quit functioning for good. If this young man still had living brain tissue, his care would likely continue. If he were deemed brain dead by the study, he would be removed from artificial life support. His body would be allowed to die, as it already would have done in any other time before the modern era of mechanical ventilators.

I walked down the hall toward the area of the radiology department designated for nuclear medicine, where radioactive isotopes are administered to patients in order to image different body parts. I slapped the square metal door opener mounted on the wall, and two wooden doors automatically opened before me. I noticed the yellow and red sign warning, "Caution: Radioactive Materials."

Common nuclear medicine studies might examine organs such as the heart, bones, or thyroid gland. Brain flow scans are less commonly ordered and performed, reserved for the most critically ill. Depending on the outcome of his study, I knew that this might be the last medical test this patient would ever have.

I rounded the corner and saw the patient being set up for his study. Only eighteen years old, he had been lively and healthy like most other teenagers, until his accident only two days prior. Unfortunately, also too often characteristic for his age group, he had been either reckless or impulsive. Entertainment on the night of his accident consisted of riding as a passenger atop an all-terrain vehicle, careening with friends along an undeveloped hillside. The intensive care unit nurse and respiratory therapist monitoring the ventilator were uncertain of the accident details, but believed that the young man had fallen off the vehicle before it proceeded to roll atop his head. He now lay motionless on a mechanical bed, with a ventilator tube passing through his mouth into his trachea. His head had sustained the brunt of his injuries. His face was heavily bruised and swollen, making his closed eyes look like two narrow slits within darkened, puffy flesh.

"I don't know if you have seen his head CT scan", the ICU nurse told me, "but I understand he had a fair amount of bleeding in his brain. His ICP keeps climbing, and we're having a harder time keeping his vital signs stable." The nurse was referring to the patient's intracranial pressure, the pressure inside his skull. That pressure was being measured by a metal probe monitor, stuck inside the patient's head like a Thanksgiving turkey thermometer. The probe reading indicated a dangerously high pressure within his skull, due to bleeding and brain swelling from the injury.

The nuclear technologist was preparing for the upcoming injection. The brain death scan relies on a simple enough concept. A small quantity of radioactive substance is injected into a vein and passes throughout the patient's blood stream. A living brain receives blood flow; a dead brain does not.

The human skull serves a wonderful purpose in protecting the brain from outside injury. However, the hard, fixed skull does not allow for much change in the volume of brain tissue. If the brain swells due to injury, and if bleeding occurs within the head, pressure builds inside the skull until the brain's arteries are squeezed shut, shunting blood away from the brain. Brain tissue is the most dependent of all the body's tissues in requiring a healthy blood supply. If its blood supply of oxygen and nutrients is interrupted for only a short period of time, the effects can be permanent, often devastating, and sometimes lethal.

The technologist tied a tourniquet around the patient's forehead, with the headband temporarily clamping blood flow in the scalp arteries, decreasing blood flow to the skin and making the study easier to interpret.

"OK, Doc, ready when you are," the technologist signaled, while the nurse and respiratory therapist both looked on.

I swallowed. "I'm ready."

He positioned the camera over the patient's head and injected the radioactive tracer in the young man's IV. Watching on the camera monitor, I saw blood pass into the carotid arteries on both sides of the neck. Some of the blood passed to the region of the patient's nose, but went no higher. No blood flowed into his brain. He was brain dead.

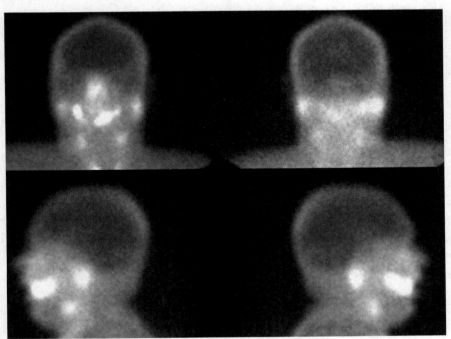

Brain death
Blood flows to the face, but the brain remains dark, having lost its blood supply.

I paused for a brief moment, before acknowledging the results aloud. Undoubtedly, the boy's parents were fearing the worst, and knew that this study might indicate the most drastic of prognoses. Yet, I knew they could never be fully prepared to receive the news they would shortly hear. After eighteen years of child rearing, their dreams for this child had ended suddenly with a senseless, tragic accident. Their investment in the future had been sabotaged.

I stared again at the motionless body. He was receiving oxygen through the ventilator tube, and his eyes were still swollen shut. I had to wonder: if the soul exists, is his trapped in that body, now void of thought and memory? Or has it already passed to its next station, leaving this protoplasm behind in a mechanically supported limbo?

The medical cascade ensued. I gave the results to the nurse and respiratory therapist. Then I called the critical care physicians and wrote a note in the patient's chart. He was transported back to intensive care, for one last family visitation prior to discontinuing the artificial support.

Perhaps the boy had been foolish and careless only for a single but critical moment, yet that moment had resulted in a permanent, devastating consequence. Nevertheless, at least once in his life he made a decision that showed some foresight and awareness of his own mortality: two years beforehand, when obtaining his driver's license, he had agreed to be an organ donor. His loved ones' grief might no longer be quite so senseless, because in one odd sense, he would exit this life as a sort of hero to others. Elsewhere at that moment, several individuals were continuing to cope with another day, their bodies ravaged by the loss of a normally functioning heart, lungs, kidneys, pancreas, or liver. Yet within several hours, they would each get a call from their respective transplant organ coordinators, notifying them of newly available, healthy organs, and a potential new lease on life.

FAMILY SECRET

In June of 2008, well-known American political commentator Tim Russert died suddenly at work from a heart attack, despite having passed a cardiac stress test only two months prior. Given the media coverage, our radiology practice saw an increase in requests for coronary artery CT studies during the aftermath. One weekday an MRI tech at one of our practice offices was talking with a CT tech, within earshot of the doctor's reading room. Elise, the doctor working that day, caught the men's attention when she unexpectedly burst into laughter. "Rob, Bill, listen to this. I'm starting a man's coronary study and was reading the history sheet. 'Reason for exam: *Because my wife made me.*'"

"That's funny," they laughed.

"It is, although who am I to talk," she admitted. "I had my husband get one a few years ago. He has some relatives with early heart disease, and I wanted the reassurance."

"So if Tim Russert had had one of these CT studies, do you think it would have made any difference?" asked Bill, the MRI tech.

"Who knows, but probably," she said. "If he had a blockage, it probably could have been discovered and treated in time."

"They're beautiful studies, if you haven't seen them," said Rob, the CT tech, who just happens to process most of the CT vascular studies for our group.

"I'm sure you would think so," Bill teased, his tone then shifting to more serious. "I wonder if I should have that done."

"Do you have risk factors?" Elise asked.

"Yes, although not the usual stuff," he explained. "My cholesterol was a little high, but it's normal now that I'm on a statin. I've never smoked, and my blood pressure is normal. But, like your husband, a lot of my relatives have had heart disease."

"How bad?" she asked.

"The worst kind," he replied. "Sudden cardiac death. Four generations now, at least, that we know of."

Her eyes widened. "What do you mean? What happened?"

"All of the men in my family have dropped dead suddenly, without any warning. No man lived past fifty-five in four generations."

"Fifty-five was the oldest?" she asked.

"Yeah, and that's the scary thing—they keep getting younger with each generation. My great-grandfather died when he was fifty-five. My grandfather died suddenly at fifty-three. My father dropped dead at forty-seven, and my brother was just shy of forty-four when he died."

"That's awful," she gasped. "Were they all on the same side of the family?"

"All on my dad's side, straight down the line."

"Do they think it was from an arrhythmia?"

"Maybe, but it's never been confirmed. They say there are people whose heart rhythm can just suddenly change from normal to dangerous, but none of my relatives was ever diagnosed with it when they were alive. Nobody ever had a pacemaker or anything. Of course my grandfather and great-grandfather died so long ago, who knows."

"That's unbelievable to have all of that in one family," she said.

Rob agreed. "Man, you need to have whatever workup you can get."

"I've had a couple of stress tests that were fine, the last one five years ago. Because of the family history, that's why my doctor keeps me on the statin for my cholesterol—he doesn't want to take any chances."

"Have you ever had your coronary arteries studied?" she asked.

"No, not directly, besides the stress tests."

"And how old are you?" she asked.

"Forty-eight," Bill said, while Rob stepped into an adjoining office to make a phone call.

"Bill, you really need to have this test done," she insisted.

"Yeah, I probably should. I'll talk to my doctor about it at my next visit."

"Definitely," she said, "only don't wait—you need to get one *now*."

Rob reentered the room. "He will," he said, smiling at Bill. "At 8:00 Monday morning, in fact. I've just called scheduling."

"What?" Bill said, surprised and looking slightly helpless. "Well, OK then, I guess it looks like I'll go ahead and have it done!"

Bill arrived for his appointment that Monday, after taking a prescribed pill to keep his heart rate relatively slow during the study, improving the quality of the pictures. He lay back and got an intravenous injection of iodine-based contrast in his arm, while the CT scanner table slid him through the large hole of the doughnut shaped machine. X-rays were beamed at his chest for a moment, and the study was done.

Rob then reconstructed the computer data to make three-dimensional pictures of Bill's coronary arteries. James, a different doctor in our group, was reading CT scans that day, and reviewed them with Bill after the study was completed.

"Your coronary arteries basically look good," James said, pointing at his computer screen while Bill looked on. "They're nearly clean—just some minimal plaque buildup."

"Good," Bill said. "That's good news. My wife will be relieved. In fact she's getting her annual mammogram today, so hopefully we'll both get a clean bill of health."

James continued looking at the pictures on his computer screen, rotating the 3-D images of Bill's heart, satisfied with the results, then briefly looked at the rest of the chest imaged. Something was quite wrong.

"Hang on a second," he said, scrolling back to review the images, then turning to face Bill directly, with a hint of concern in his voice. "How do you feel?"

"Until you mentioned that, just fine," Bill smiled. "Why, do you see something?"

"Give me a minute," James said, disbelieving what was right before his eyes, in the man right in front of him. He clicked through the images again, but the interpretation did not change. "Are you breathing OK? Any shortness of breath, or chest pain?"

"No," Bill denied.

"Have you taken any recent trip—been on a plane, or stuck in a car a long time?"

"No—why? What do you see?"

"You've got multiple pulmonary emboli." James read the confusion and disbelief on Bill's face. "The arteries supplying blood to your lungs are full of blood clots."

"Are you sure?" Bill asked.

"Yes. Here they are," James pointed to the images. "There's no question. But you should be really sick. Most people with this much blood clot have symptoms. Are you sure you feel OK?"

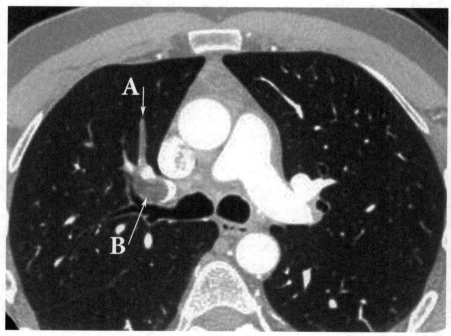

Pulmonary embolism
The dark gray areas (A&B) represent blood clots in
some of the arteries that supply blood to his lungs.

"Yeah," Bill said.

"There's got to be some mistake. Let me call the CT control room—is it possible they could have mixed your study up with someone else, and gotten the names switched?"

No error had occurred. The pictures belonged to Bill.

Rob, the coworker who had scheduled and subsequently processed Bill's study, was across the hall and could hear the conversation. He retrieved a pulse oximeter, a small machine that checks the amount of oxygen in the bloodstream by sliding a thimble-shaped device over a fingernail, emitting a red laser beam that measures the percentage of red blood cells that are carrying oxygen. Bill's level was 95%.

"That level sounds fine, right?" he asked.

"It's pretty good," James hesitated, "but it's not quite normal for a healthy person." Rob checked his own to test the accuracy of the machine; his reading was 99%.

"That's normal," James said. "Bill, I think you need to get admitted to the hospital. I'm going to telephone the pulmonologist on call."

"Is it that serious?" Bill asked. "I don't feel bad, honestly."

It was indeed serious. The heart pumps oxygen-poor blood from the body's veins to the lungs, where the blood binds oxygen and releases carbon dioxide. If the arteries to the lungs contain clots, the blood flow to the lungs is partially blocked. If enough blockage occurs, the condition can be fatal. Regardless of how much the person tries to breathe, oxygen cannot get from the lungs into the bloodstream. It's like drowning in the open air.

Bill had no idea anything was wrong until the discovery was made, during a study designed to look for a different problem altogether. "Can you all call my wife? She's having her mammogram over at the breast center."

Bill's wife had just completed getting her mammogram when the call came through. She waited in the x-ray room while her mammogram was being checked by the radiologist at that office. Moments later the x-ray tech and the radiologist walked in, both of them looking worried.

"I don't like that look on your face," Bill's wife said. "What did you find?"

"On you, nothing," the radiologist replied. "Your mammogram is fine. But your husband is getting sent to the hospital as we speak."

I saw Bill later that day at the hospital, where I was working.

He had more radiology studies ordered to see why he was forming blood clots. An ultrasound of his legs showed no clot in his leg veins, the most common site where blood clots form. An additional CT of his abdomen and pelvis showed no clot there either, nor any tumor, or any other disease that can predispose someone to form blood clots. The reason for the clots was a mystery.

"This is an amazing story," I told him as he reiterated the events of the day.

"Tell me about it. I thought I was fine, just being cautious, and now I've landed in the hospital for a couple of days, until they can get my blood thinned."

"You're still feeling OK?" I asked again.

"Just fine, normal. I took my son to the pool yesterday and was swimming underwater. I don't feel short of breath, and don't have any pain."

The next day I briefly stopped by Bill's hospital room. He still felt fine. His wife and their ten-year-old son were by his side.

"Bill, I've got to ask—before they started the blood thinners, did they draw blood for some tests to check your clotting function?"

"They took all kinds of blood, a bunch of tubes," he confirmed.

"Good. You've got a good pulmonologist in charge of your case, and it sounds like she's doing everything she can think of to get to the bottom of this. You realize that this could explain the family history you've got, if one of those tests comes back abnormal."

"Yeah, although she said it's not very common."

"No, but neither is your family history, fortunately. So besides those normal stress tests you mentioned, there's been no other study to look for an arrhythmia?"

"Actually, yes. A couple of years ago I wore a Holter monitor for at least 24 hours, and it didn't reveal anything significant."

His son, an affable kid with a dry sense of humor, slightly teased his dad like a typical ten-year-old would do. "I won't say that dad is *weird*, but I could have told you he was kind of different," the boy slightly smiled, unable to hide his more genuine affection and admiration. Bill and his wife smiled back.

"Just think, son," I said, "depending on how your dad's lab

tests turn out, you may get the chance to have all kinds of blood drawn, too."

"Great," he rolled his eyes.

"And of course your dad will need to be waited on a lot while he's recovering at home. Maybe you could give him some good foot rubs."

"Not me!" The boy made a face while his parents continued to smile.

Bill got discharged after a couple of nights at the hospital. He has done well on blood thinners for over a decade since, now having lived longer than any of the men in his paternal lineage for at least five generations. I was certain that a rare hereditary clotting disorder would be found to explain his blood clots and his family history of sudden death. Time and technology still point in the direction of that hypothesis, but they have not yet revealed a final verdict by name. Blood tests that detect several known cellular and protein clotting disorders all came back normal. Of course, these disorders have not always been known to scientists, and others are still yet unknown, or incompletely understood. What is clear from Bill's CT is that he readily, and silently, without symptoms or warning, forms blood clots that lodge in his lungs. The presumed but still undetermined clotting disorder that has likely wreaked havoc on Bill's family for generations now appears halted in its tracks with improved anticoagulation medicines, which no one knew he needed until he had that CT scan, demonstrating the silent but potentially fatal abnormality.

We are reminded again of the power of imaging, its ability to solve medical mysteries, and of the humbling fact that we never know what secrets one may discover once we start looking.

SECTION III: THE MORE UNUSUAL

L ike the stories in the preceding sections, these chapters also describe intriguing, revelatory glimpses of people and their lives, through their imaging studies. However, the stories selected for this section contain elements of a less common nature, whether it be an uncommon diagnosis, unexpected behavior, or other surprise circumstance. In addition to the diagnoses described, these vignettes further explore the nuances of communication and perception sometimes required in the field of medicine—even for doctors who are not the primary care physicians.

The final chapter in this section, "Spared," deserves additional commentary. It has taken several forms, with changes in text and title, but I ultimately decided to let it stand on its own, short but poignant. Its preface is this: sometimes coincidence can have profound, life-altering impact. In fact, I have seen enough cases over the years to recognize that coincidence is not so rare as we think it is, although it is still nearly unbelievable each time it happens, and profound for each individual affected.

Some examples: a woman feels a lump in one breast, prompting her to get a mammogram she would otherwise have put off. The lump she feels turns out to be a benign cyst; but the mammogram finds an early-stage cancer in a different part of the same breast, or on the opposite side, and she is cured.

Pancreatic cancer is notorious for being silent and asymptomatic until it has already metastasized to an incurable status. Yet at least three times in my career have I seen patients get CT scans for abdominal pain (twice for appendicitis, once for a kidney stone), and a pancreatic cancer was discovered. In all three cases, the tumors were removed before spreading. Other cancers, like kidney cancer or lymphoma, are even more commonly discovered as an unexpected finding when still relatively small, when patients have scans performed for other reasons.

Sometimes someone else benefits from the situation. I once performed a study on a healthy young woman to look at the blood supply to her kidneys. Her sister had gone into renal failure, and my patient was going to donate a kidney to keep her sister alive and off of dialysis.

"I had a miscarriage only a few months ago," she explained, "and at the time I was so upset. But if I had remained pregnant, I wouldn't be able to undergo these x-ray tests now to give my sister a kidney. Things really have a strange way of working out sometimes."

Indeed they do.

IN THE DARK

Another day during internship, I was paged to the emergency room to admit a woman to the hospital. She was a heavy smoker in her late sixties who had not seen a doctor for years. For two weeks the woman had become progressively weaker at home, also losing her vision and becoming incontinent. Only when she became unable to walk did she finally succumb to her family's request that she see a doctor. Given the condition into which she had deteriorated, and the fact that the woman had no doctor of her own, her family brought her to the emergency room.

Fearing that she had suffered a stroke, the emergency room physicians ordered a CT scan of the woman's head upon her arrival. The CT scan did not show a stroke; it showed that she had metastatic cancer in her brain. A chest x-ray taken afterward showed a sizable lung mass, consistent with the primary cancer.

The medical resident supervising me accompanied me into the woman's emergency room cubicle. The woman's debilitation made her look old beyond her years, as she stared glassy eyed at the ceiling, only semi-aware of what was going on around her. I stood in the light and gently squeezed her hand as I introduced myself.

"Ma'am, I'm Dr. Ruff, and this is Dr. Patel," I gestured toward the young dark-haired woman by my side. "We're going to admit you to the hospital here, but we need to ask you a few questions and examine you for a few minutes."

A short, younger woman with brown hair, glasses, and pale skin stepped in from behind the curtain. She looked anxious.

"I'm sorry, I just went to make a phone call. I'm her daughter."

"No need to apologize," I said. "We were just explaining to

your mother that we do want to admit her to the hospital. I was just getting ready to explain what the CT scan and chest x-ray showed. I know she must be worn out and a bit confused from the events of the day, so I am relieved you are here, although I regret the news is not good."

The woman's daughter, looking more anxious, stopped me. "Could I talk to you all outside for just a minute?" she asked.

Dr. Patel and I followed her through the curtain surrounding the woman's bed, and continued following her nearly twenty feet, where we were no longer in earshot to her mother.

"I really need to tell you all that my mother would not want to know any bad news. I know it can't be good, and you can tell me whatever she's got, but please don't tell her."

After a brief but pensive pause, Dr. Patel spoke first. "Normally if patients are of sound mind, they make their medical decisions themselves. It would be unusual to share that information with anyone else but withhold it from the patient, as long as she is able to participate in her medical decisions."

"She'd rather I handle it, I'm sure of it," the daughter replied.

Dr. Patel and I hesitated to speak as we studied the young woman and processed her request.

"Most patients cope better when they know what they're up against," I explained. "It's tough enough to be sick, but worse to feel bad and not know why. Patients typically tell us that they would rather be told the truth than be left with their fear of the unknown."

"Trust me, I'm certain that she would not want to know. I can't bear the waiting any longer. What do you all think is wrong with her?" she asked.

My resident let me do the talking. "We're sorry to tell you that your mother has a mass in her lung, and several lesions in her brain. You never know until you get a sample of tissue and can have it analyzed under a microscope, but the CT and x-ray do not look good. We are afraid that your mom has cancer, probably lung cancer that has spread to her brain."

The young woman raised trembling hands to cover her quivering mouth, and we motioned her to a nearby chair.

"I was afraid of this," she said. "She has been doing so poorly,

I just knew that it was something serious. She hasn't seen a doctor in years. She is afraid of them, afraid of hearing bad news. How bad is it?"

"It's pretty bad," I said. "If it's confirmed to be a metastatic cancer, as we suspect, there is very little hope for cure, particularly given the spread to her brain. Her brain also shows signs of mild swelling from the tumors, likely making her symptoms worse. We could give her some medicine to try to decrease the swelling, but it may not help that much. And once we get tissue diagnosis, we can talk about other treatment options like possible chemotherapy, but again, the benefit at this point might be really limited."

"This is a lot of information at once. We are sorry to be the bearers of such bad news," Dr. Patel said, reaching out to hold the daughter's hands.

"It is awful news, but there's no other way than to say it," the daughter said. "Thank you for being honest with me, but please don't tell my mother that you think she has cancer."

Dr. Patel and I looked at each other. "Let's go check on your mother together for a moment," I suggested. "I won't say anything right now, and if I get the feeling from your mom that she genuinely doesn't want to know, then we can talk about it."

The three of us went back into the cubicle together. The woman was lying on the stretcher, breathing quietly with her eyes closed. "Ma'am, we're back, the doctors who are going to bring you into the hospital. Your daughter is here and wants to say *hi*."

The woman opened her eyes, but they stared without focus toward the ceiling. The daughter grabbed her mother's hand. "Mom, I'm with you."

"You've got a very caring daughter who is concerned about you," I said. "We got a chance to talk with her for just a minute, but we really haven't talked to you about what we think is going on. Would you like to know?" I asked.

"No," the woman said, shaking her head, still staring at the ceiling with a vacant expression.

"So you don't have a problem if we talk to your daughter, but not to you?"

"You can talk to her," she said, a detached look of fear developing on her face.

"But you don't want to know what's going on yourself?" we asked once more.

"No, no," she shook her head, still fearful, unable to focus on our faces.

The next morning we presented the woman's case to the rest of the team at morning rounds. No one on the team had any ethical objection to withholding the diagnosis from the patient, as she and her daughter were in agreement with the arrangement. Dr. Rodriguez, the attending physician in charge of our team, encouraged us to look into the possibility of a lung biopsy with the radiologists.

After rounds, I took the patient's chest x-ray and head CT to one of the radiologists. "You may have read this yesterday, I'm not sure," I began, "but this is a woman with a mass in her lung, plus several in her brain, likely metastatic lung cancer. I'll be honest, she probably doesn't want anything done about it anyway, and doesn't even want to know what's wrong with her. Nevertheless, we would at least like to confirm the diagnosis. Do you think you could get a piece of tissue for us?"

"We ought to be able to biopsy the lung mass by CT," he said.

"That would be great, thanks. I'll order the biopsy."

He did the biopsy the next day. The tissue showed lung cancer.

In the meantime, we were trying to figure out what to do with the woman who did not want to face her own illness. We were not doing much for her in the hospital, but she was clearly too sick to send home. She ate and drank very little, getting progressively weaker each day. She stayed drowsy but was at least somewhat lucid when we roused her.

"She is really pitiful," I updated Dr. Patel and Dr. Rodriguez. "She can't get out of bed at all, and I think she is nearly blind. She has got to be scared, not knowing what the heck is going on, but she still refuses to be informed about her condition."

"Denial can be a powerful defense mechanism," Rodriguez said.

Every day the woman's daughter was at the hospital. She never failed to thank us for all we were doing for her mother, even though there was very little we could do for her.

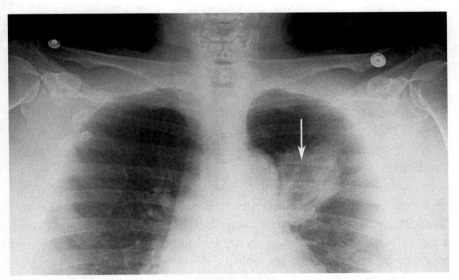

Lung cancer
Mass in the upper left lung on chest x-ray. Biopsy revealed lung cancer.

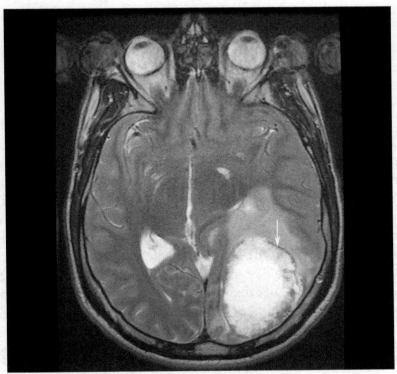

Lung cancer metastasis to the brain on MRI

"I still haven't told your mother that she has cancer, and don't see the need to do so. You were right. She really doesn't want to face it."

"No, but I sure do appreciate all you've done to try to keep her comfortable. All of our family does."

"Not at all. At least she doesn't seem to be in any pain right now. If the need arises, we could give her some pain medicine."

"If she needs any, although she's never been fond of taking medicines."

"I believe that. I need to ask you about a couple of other things. If her condition continues to worsen, how aggressive do you think she would want her treatment to be? What if her heart were to stop, of if she were to stop breathing? Do you think she would want to be resuscitated, including CPR or a ventilator?"

"No, definitely not," her daughter said. "She would absolutely hate to be kept alive on a machine. I can't image anything worse for her. She's always made it very clear that she would not want to be kept alive artificially."

"Would that include being fed by a tube?" I asked.

"Yes it would. I am certain she would not want that, and no one in the family would want her to suffer like that."

The daughter continued to make things surprisingly easy for us, given the fact that there was little we could do for the woman, and no real ethical dilemma regarding her comfort care. It was clear that this woman was never going to go home, and it became clearer that the hospital was not the best place for her to stay, certainly not from a financial perspective. We enlisted the support of a hospital social worker in order to find the woman a bed at a local nursing home facility where hospice care could be provided. Unfortunately, no bed was available. Because this woman had not seen a doctor in so long, she was still in the process of being registered for Medicare benefits, and still qualifying for Medicaid. While the bureaucratic process continued at its expected pace, the patient continued to lie in her hospital bed and deteriorate daily.

The social worker saw me and Dr. Patel at the nurse's station one afternoon. "I may have a lead on one facility, but it's going to be a while," she said. "I'll see what I can do and let you know if I have any luck."

"Thanks," we said.

After a combined time lapse of about two weeks, it was clear that the woman would soon die. Although I was still more or less comfortable withholding the information of her diagnosis from her, given the consistency of her and her family's wishes, it was still awkward trying to comfort her on one level, as we were never able to tell her directly that she was dying, and that we knew why. In retrospect, she had to know, too, at least on some level.

By this point she was no longer eating at all, and she drifted further and further into a steady trance, from which it became harder to rouse her. The social worker still had no word about getting the patient transferred to another facility. We decided that it would probably be too disruptive for the dying patient to move her, and perhaps too unsettling for the family to watch her get shipped out of the hospital with only a few days to live.

I saw the daughter again the next day, standing outside of her mother's room. "We don't have any new news today," I told her. "Your mother is obviously less alert now, but she still seems comfortable and in no pain as far as we can tell."

"No, she does seem comfortable at least," the young woman said, lifting her glasses just enough to wipe a small tear from the corner of one eye.

"You may remember that we talked about ten days ago about the possibility of having her transferred to a nursing home. I'd say that at this point it's probably not worth the bother. No one can say how much longer she'll live, but we don't think it's going to be more than a few days."

"We all didn't think so either, as poorly as she's doing now. But we do want to thank you all again so much for all of your help. You've been so kind throughout all of this."

"You're more than welcome. We're just sorry that there wasn't more that we could do."

I checked on the dying woman every day. She lay peacefully in her silent room, with the curtains drawn and the lights barely lit. In her last days, she either slept or stared blankly toward the ceiling, not really responding to people, unable to focus on anyone or anything in her exterior world.

After the woman died, I saw her daughter one last time outside her mother's door. She held back her tears enough to thank us one more time.

I went to the nurse's station to write a final note in the patient's chart, after pronouncing the woman dead. I handed the chart to the secretary, a friendly, middle-aged black woman.

"This patient just passed away," I said. "Everything is signed and ready to go. Her daughter is here, if you need any further information from the family. Bless her heart, the daughter is still thanking us, even though we didn't do much. Her gratitude is amazing."

"Don't be too amazed," the secretary told me, picking up the patient's chart. "I know that family, and if you had any idea how much trouble that girl has caused her poor mother over the years, you'd see this in a whole new light. She might hang around at the end acting like she's taking care of her mother, but that doesn't change how she treated that lady all this time."

I did not ask her to elaborate, and still have no clue what she meant.

FRACTURED

Sue, a radiology nurse at the city hospital during residency, stopped me in the hallway and warned me about our next patient.

"The young woman you all are doing a myelogram on this morning is such a sad case," she began. "You simply won't believe all the bad things that have happened to her. She's in the room with Anita from CT, and is going to need some extra hand holding, the poor thing."

With that warning, I prepared to meet the unfortunate thirty-year old woman who had already had neck surgery a year before for a bad disk. The surgery presumably must have been less than successful, since she was already back for more tests.

I was not, however, prepared for what I found. Immediately upon entering the windowless hospital examination room, I wondered why this woman was wearing sunglasses inside.

The nurse and CT tech looked on as I introduced myself, reaching out to shake the young woman's hand. She extended her arm with hesitation, giving me a grip that felt considerably weaker than her firmly toned body looked capable of giving. Her brown hair was long and straight, framing an expressionless visible lower half of her face, the upper half obscured by her large shades. She also wore a removable brace on her left forearm, the kind one could find at a pharmacy, and a drugstore knee brace on one leg.

Her doctor's order indicated that the young woman had had two neck vertebrae fused the previous year. Surprisingly, she was already complaining of recurrent tingling and numbness in both arms. Her neurosurgeon ordered the study called a CT myelogram to evaluate the nerve roots in her neck. Still in residency, I would be

95

performing the myelogram under supervision.

"I'm sorry to hear that you're still having trouble, after going through your surgery last year," I began.

"Yeah, it's really awful," she began, speaking very slowly, deliberately, taking a great deal of effort. "I just don't think I will ever be right again." She sounded really tired, with surprising pauses and occasional emphasis for added effect. "I used to be a fitness instructor. I sure couldn't do that now. I've been out of work for a long time, and don't know what I'm going to do." She sighed. "I applied for disability, but my case is still pending, and those people in the government office don't seem to want to help. They just try to wear you down, until you give up, because it's too much for someone who's weak and sick to try to go up against a big office like that..."

"I'm sorry about that," I said, wanting to get to the root of the medical problem she was there for that day. She did not come across as assertive but rambled in her story, as if trying to evoke sympathy. I had still heard nothing about her nerve symptoms. "Let me ask about your current situation, so we can talk about this procedure today. Did your neck surgery give you relief initially?"

She took a breath, and exhaled slowly. "Well, it started like this. What happened was my boyfriend threw me down a flight of stairs, and hurt my neck," she continued in her slow, deliberate cadence. "It was in the stairwell of our apartment building. Not one of the neighbors called the police at first. They said later that they didn't know anything had happened, but I don't see how they could have missed the screaming, it was so painful."

The nurse and CT tech looked on sympathetically, shaking their heads while the young woman spoke. Yet the more she did speak, the more I felt that she was trying to manipulate us.

"Anyway, I guess one neighbor eventually must have called the cops, and they arrested my ex, but it's tough living with a restraining order when you can't..."

"I am really sorry that that happened to you," I tried to comfort, "but for your test today, I need to ask you more specifically about your current symptoms."

She sighed, frustrated, dejected. "I am just trying to tell you that I was fine, until he punched me, broke my jaw, then threw me down the stairs and left me for dead. I cracked some ribs and passed out..."

Her jaw line looked fine currently, with no scar.

"I feel like I am having a little trouble connecting with you," I said. "I can't even see you, really. Would you mind taking off your sunglasses for a moment?"

The request upset her slightly, as she searched for reasons not to show her face. "Uh, well, uh, it's just that these lights in here..."

"They're not that bright, really," I assured. "I don't like strong lights either, but I don't think these will bother you. Just raise your glasses for a minute if you would, so I can at least see what you look like."

She began lifting her non-injured, non-splinted right arm toward her face, grimacing and beginning to moan as if she had been asked to lift a sack of bricks with an extended pinky. Eventually she put her fingers on the sunglasses frame, and with great effort, slowly lifted the lenses so that I could barely see her eyes from beneath the rims, as if she were peering from a cave.

"Uh, it's just, so, um,..." she muttered as she started to let the glasses slide back onto her nose.

"Don't worry about it, if it bothers you that much," I said, suspecting a great more was behind her need for those sunglasses than just light sensitivity. "Let's get back to the myelogram. Have you ever had a study like this before?"

"I've had CT scans before, after I was mugged once. A guy jumped me in a parking lot, and gave me a concussion, and scraped my face against the asphalt. They brought me here in an ambulance..."

"When was that?"

"Well, it must have been four years ago, because that was around the time that my old boyfriend..." she said. The nurse and tech looked on in sympathy, but my suspicions were on red alert.

"Okay. Have you ever had a lumbar puncture? A spinal tap?"

"No, let's see. No, I've had a lot of other stuff, but no, I don't think so," she thought aloud.

"Have you ever had any children?" I asked, thinking of an epidural.

"No," she replied, her shortest answer yet. "But I am worried about that, because I am already in so much pain from these fractures."

"What fractures?" I asked.

"Well, you see what happened was, I was getting off of a city bus just last week, and because of the trouble with my neck, I can't turn my head well, and the driver was being really impatient, and wasn't waiting for me to get down the stairs and step off onto the curb, and so he started to move a little bit when I fell, and I hit the sidewalk really hard. All these people were standing around me, and somebody called an ambulance, and they brought me here, and the x-rays showed that I broke my arm, and have a hairline fracture in my leg."

I looked at the drugstore braces that she wore. "They didn't put a cast on you?"

"No, this is all they gave me. I hope these heal up okay on account of that. But they definitely told me in the emergency room that the bones were broken on the x-rays."

The nurse and CT tech continued to look on, empathetic listening to her tragic story. She was a sad figure indeed, clearly needy—but her tale was becoming less fathomable the more I observed, and the more she spoke.

"Anyway, because of the pain I'm having in my bones, it's going to be really hard for me to do this test, to lie back on that table, but I'll try. I know I have to, so I'll go through with it as best as I can."

"Excuse me for just a minute," I said. "I need to check on something and will be right back." Sue and Anita looked at me, puzzled that I would suddenly walk out like that.

I left the room, went straight to a computer terminal, and looked up the patient's records. She had indeed been seen recently in the emergency room, just like she said, but the rest of her story was quite different. The x-ray images had shone clear truth onto the murky, deceptive story she was trying to spin.

Her x-rays were read as normal. They showed no fracture. The emergency doctors knew this, found nothing serious on her examination, and released her in satisfactory condition, with no brace or splint. The woman had obtained those herself, after she was discharged.

Her x-ray jacket was on the counter outside of the room where we were talking. I held the films up to a light and also saw no fractures.

I walked back into the room, intent on taking charge of the situation. "You said you were treated here last week for your recent injuries."

Immediately she shifted in her seat, not grimacing at all when she moved the leg with the brace. "Well, yeah, yes..."

"Not treated anywhere else?"

"No, no, I was here, it was right here, at this hospital," she insisted.

"OK, I know, because I just looked up your records. But there's a bit of a problem here."

"I, uh, I don't understand," she stammered. "What, I mean..."

"I looked at your x-rays, and the reports," I explained. "Your x-rays were normal. They did not show that you broke those bones, like you said."

The nurse and CT tech were looking wide-eyed at me, first surprised at the changed tone in my voice, then more surprised at the information itself. All three of us then stared at her in unison. Still wearing her sunglasses, she turned her head, further avoiding our collective gaze, caught defenseless in her own game.

"But, oh, uh, I don't understand," she lightly wailed, raising her arms in the air in helplessness, further stammering, shifting in her seat again, trying to deny. The nurse went to her.

"There are plenty of things I don't understand. We're trying to help you, but that would be a whole lot easier to do if you could give me a straight answer."

Again she moaned, lifting her sunglasses only just enough so that she could rub her fingers over her eyes. I saw no tears through the darkened façade. She was trying to deceive and mask on so many levels, but the x-rays told me everything that she would not. Caught in her act, she was visibly frustrated.

"I don't understand," she muttered, "oh, I just want this to be over..."

"The study will be over sooner, and you can get out of here sooner, if you just level with us and stay on track. Let's talk about this procedure—why you're having it, and a few small risks I need to inform you about to get your consent to proceed."

"I'm trying," she moaned. "I'm in pain."

"Again, we're trying to help you. For that to happen, you've got to try a little harder to stay focused here. I'm sorry for any troubles you've had outside of here, truly, but if we're going to do this test that your doctor wants you to have, you've got to answer a few questions."

Eventually, finally, she subdued herself and complied with our instructions for the study. Her lumbar puncture and contrast injection were uneventful, and her CT scan was normal. Whatever her problem was, there was no visible evidence that it had anything to do with her nerve roots after neck surgery. Objectively the operation looked to have been a complete success.

Her course after the CT myelogram procedure, however, was another story.

I was back in the reading room, trying to get through a stack of studies that had accumulated while the myelogram consent process had taken so much longer than usual. I also had to prepare for a couple of other procedures besides hers, now behind schedule. Sue, the nurse, came to see me. "Our patient with the myelogram is now complaining of a severe headache."

"Did you give her any acetaminophen? I wrote for some, just in case."

"I offered it to her," she said, "but she didn't want that."

"Oh joy," I sighed, having seen behavior like this before.

"She's on a stretcher in recovery. Maybe you could take a look at her."

I summoned the professor who had done the myelogram with me. "I'd appreciate it if you'd come with me for this one. I may need reinforcement, not to mention a witness."

The young woman was the only patient at that moment in the tranquil recovery area, lying on a stretcher in the corner. The ceiling lights were dim, and she still had her sunglasses on.

Quietly we approached her bedside and spoke. "How are you feeling?"

"Please leave," she whispered, barely audible.

"The nurse told me that you weren't feeling well, and we came to check on you."

"Please leave," she whispered again.

"Where do you hurt?"

"Everywhere," she said. "I've got a migraine."

"Is that why the light is bothering you? A migraine?"

"Yes," she said softly. "Your study hurt me. You never said that I would hurt like this. It's awful."

"Actually, we did warn you that some people do feel a headache afterward, if you remember, but it's usually not this bad. Then again, you were bothered by the lights before we even got started. If it's a migraine you've got, we could get you something for it. Have you ever had Imitrex? The injectable form is fast acting—I could order some from the pharmacy."

"No, it won't help," she said softly lightly shaking her head. "It won't work."

"What do you mean, have you tried it before?" I asked.

"I've tried everything. It's no use. I'll need something else," she whispered again.

"I don't want to leave you with an untreated migraine if we can do something about it. They're no fun, I know."

She raised up on her elbows and turned her head toward us. "You have no idea how I've suffered with headaches over the years," she blurted, her voice suddenly above normal volume. "I've tried everything. Pills, it doesn't matter, they don't do anything. They just don't work on me."

"Have you ever seen a neurologist?"

She ignored the question. "In fact, I remember only one time when a doctor was kind enough to give me some medicine that helped take the pain away."

I had a feeling what was coming. "And what medicine was that?"

"Well, you see, I had been in this car wreck, and felt so bad from all kinds of injuries..."

"And they gave you?"

"....so anyway, I was laid up, really bruised and sore all over, and the headaches were just intense," she whispered.

"The medicine," I said.

"...and nobody would give me anything to feel better, because they didn't care, except finally for this one doctor, who was nice enough..."

"Please, tell me: which medicine are you asking for?" I pleaded.

"...so finally somebody took some pity when they saw how bad I was doing..."

"Look, you could answer this question in one word. I *know* you know the name of the drug, so in *one word*, please, just say it."

"What I am *trying* to *tell* you," she blurted out loudly, "is that the only thing that has ever helped is *Demerol*."

"Demerol," I reiterated, flatly. "No way. I get migraines myself. People shouldn't need a narcotic like that for a migraine. It's not what you use to treat..."

"Now you look here," she raised her voice, sitting up abruptly and pointing her finger in the air. "I have come in here and done everything that you all told me to do, had a needle stuck in my back, desperate to do anything to get some help, because nobody, it seems, wants to help me get any better, and I guess you all are no different. You promised me that this wouldn't hurt, only now you have made it worse," she fumed.

"You're getting your energy back," I said, noticing the sudden transition in her tone. "That's a good sign. Maybe your headache is getting better."

She paused briefly, then fired back, "I've had to keep going to survive. You have no idea what I've been through, or what kind of pain I have to put up with every day, day in and day out. Which is why it makes me that much madder when medical people won't listen to you and don't want to help you."

"I don't want you or anybody else to suffer. I'd actually love for you to feel better and get some help, really."

She lay back, her voice softening like before. "Not if you don't give me anything for pain. Please leave."

"I'm going to ask the nurse to get you some acetaminophen, and some water. Let's let you rest and see if you feel any better."

She sat back up abruptly. "I am *telling* you, that's not going to *work* on me," she said. "I'm different."

"Oh, I could believe that, sincerely. But let's start with that and see how you feel."

Eventually, the patient was able, and willing, to leave, with no narcotics given. After her discharge, the nurse and CT tech approached me together.

"She was unbelievable," Anita said. "She had us fooled, at first anyway."

"I know. Which isn't to say that she's not feeling some of the symptoms she claims—even though we can't prove it, or find any valid reason for it."

"You didn't see anything abnormal on her myelogram?" Sue asked.

"No, it looked good. The only thing I saw abnormal was the patient in the room, not the images on the scan."

"I wonder what she's really after, and how long she's been acting this way?" Anita pondered.

"It's got to be more than just drug seeking," Sue commented. "She's willing to go through with the procedures."

"She's a tough nut to crack," I agreed. "I read her chart more after the procedure, and her neurologist not only gave her a psych referral, he personally walked her to the psychiatry department to make sure she scheduled an appointment. We're not the first people to recognize that she could benefit from some mental health, but we might be the first to actually prove it with a couple of normal bone films. We tried, but let's face it: what she needs right now is a good psychiatrist, not another x-ray."

ABUSED

The office radiology practice had been busier than usual for a winter Thursday afternoon. It was my first year in private practice after residency and fellowship training, and days like this one tested my ability to do thorough work while keeping up with the volume. The barium cases took longer than expected. Many children and adults came in for chest x-rays, as it was the height of the cold and flu season. I also needed time to review a mammogram with an elderly woman who had a new abnormality that could be cancerous and would require a biopsy. In addition, a woman with worsening abdominal and back pain had an unexpected 10 cm aortic aneurysm on a CT scan that afternoon, roughly five times the normal diameter, so large that I arranged to have her immediately admitted to the hospital, fearing that the severely dilated artery could burst at any time.

The films were piled high on my counter, with no room on the light boxes in the reading office, yet Jane, the x-ray technologist, returned and interrupted me with a chest x-ray on a child only four months old. "Can you read this one next please? This baby has a cough, like most of the people who have walked in here today. The doctor wants to make sure that this girl doesn't have pneumonia, and wants us to call with a wet reading." Jane is a delight, someone who works hard but likes to have fun in the process. She smiled as her voice lowered and adopted the pretend tone of a seasoned expert. "My professional opinion is that she does not have pneumonia, sir."

I put the film on the light box in front of me, glimpsed briefly, and agreed with her mock interpretation. The film showed signs of a mild viral bronchitis, but no pneumonia. Yet as I completed visually inspecting the film before taking it down, my heart rate began to increase. An unsuspected but extremely important abnormality lay right before me on the film. The child had six consecutive rib fractures on one side. The fractures were not recent. Calcium deposits at the fracture sites indicated that they had been healing for several weeks.

I knew what condition I had probably discovered, but I almost tried to talk myself out of the diagnosis, not wanting to believe what I was seeing. Unfortunately, the abnormalities and their implications could not be denied. As my pulse continued to increase, my mind began to recall important lessons from earlier training regarding childhood fractures.

A child this age, not yet even able to crawl, would not be able to inflict significant injury upon herself. Unless she had been in a recent accident, this baby had likely been squeezed or hit hard enough by someone to break her ribs. I suspected and feared that I was looking at my first case of newly discovered child abuse.

"Who brought her in, her mother?" I asked.

"Both parents," she answered. "Why?"

"Keep the baby and the parents here," I said, showing her the findings. "This kid has some healing rib fractures, right here, and I need to let the doctor know. We may need to get some more x-rays."

I called the pediatrician immediately, and conveyed the film findings. "Was there anything suspicious on your physical exam?"

"No, I just ordered the chest x-ray to make sure there was no pneumonia. She has no bruises. Are you certain of the findings?"

"No question, they're real," I confirmed.

"That's very interesting. Could you get a complete skeletal survey while they're still there?"

He was asking for a series of x-ray films of the child's skull, limbs, spine, and pelvis, routinely done to evaluate the rest of the bones if child abuse is suspected. We needed to see if the child had any other fractures, of either the same or different ages as the ones I had already seen. Such findings would further raise suspicion for deliberately inflicted trauma.

Knowing that I should try to keep reading other patients' films until the skeletal survey was complete, I had a hard time focusing, given my preoccupation with the case at hand. Jane returned moments later, having recruited a second technologist, Amy, to help hold the baby for the series of x-rays. The two women revealed that the parents were beginning to act strangely.

"Something is definitely weird about that father," Jane opined. "He insists on cradling that baby in his arms in between each film we take. He's not just protective, he's being overly doting. He almost won't hand her over for the next film after each exposure."

Amy agreed. "That's not all. When the mother gathered that there was no pneumonia, but still something wrong, and that the pediatrician wanted more x-rays, she immediately called her father on her cell phone, and asked him to drive over here to our office as soon as possible. That's just not normal behavior, unless they know something's going on."

"Anyway, the films should be out in a few minutes," Jane said.

I could not concentrate on the accumulating pile of other patients' films. I knew that it was not fair to pass judgment prematurely on these people, but my suspicions, curiosity, and anxiety would not go away. The consequences were too serious. Finally, Jane and Amy returned with the awaited bone films. The child's skull, pelvis, spine, and legs appeared normal. One of her arms also appeared fine. Yet when I looked at the opposite arm, there were signs suspicious of a fracture at the child's wrist. Fractures in this location, especially at this age, typically result from an adult twisting a child's arm in a fit of rage. There was very little doubt now that this child was being physically abused.

Again, I telephoned the pediatrician, informing him of the suspected wrist fracture as well. He thanked me for calling, told me that he would look into the matter officially, and asked me to send the x-rays and the family back over to his office. I gave the films my final review, found nothing else, and began dictating the report.

The more certain I was of the diagnosis, the more confused I became by the questions racing through my head. Who was hurting this child? Was it the father? The mother? Was it a babysitter, or a sibling? Did anyone else know about the abuse? Does the perpetrator realize that the trauma inflicted was severe enough to break bones? Does he or she believe that the truth will never be discovered? What kind of person would do this? And what drives a person to lose control of his anger and inflict trauma upon a defenseless baby?

A moment I had dreaded, yet also anticipated with fascination, broke the silence in my dark reading room, interrupting the chain of internal questions that preoccupied me. "The child's mother would like to speak with you," Jane informed me, looking serious and cautious. I stepped out into the hall, met the mother, and motioned her to a quiet corner to discuss her child's x-ray findings.

"Thank you for your patience while we got all the x-rays on your baby here."

"Take your time and do whatever you need." Her face showed a mixture of worry, sadness, confusion, and fear. "I'm just really concerned about whatever you must have seen."

I studied her expression. Did she already know that I might be seeing signs of abuse? I tried to dismiss any suspicion and focused on the discussion with her.

"I'm sure you must be worried," I replied honestly, although not sure what she was most worried about. "Let me explain what we've found. The chest x-ray did not show any sign of pneumonia, which is obviously good. However, your daughter has six rib fractures that look like they're probably a few weeks old. Has she been in any kind of accident recently, like a car crash?"

"No, not that I can think of," she replied.

"Perhaps she was dropped accidentally?" I suggested. "Maybe by a babysitter, or an older sibling?"

"No, not that I'm aware of." Her look of worry remained.

"Is there any history of childhood bone disease in the family?" I asked.

"No," she shook her head.

"As a matter of routine, whenever we see unexplained fractures in an infant, we take the series of x-rays that we just got, in order to look for any other fractures. The rib fractures are definite, but I'm also worried that she probably has a small fracture at her left wrist as well," I stated, directly but calmly. "That one is more subtle, but I do think it's real."

She nodded, but looked more confused. Her lips quivered

slightly, and her eyes were wide open with disbelief, but she remained engaged in the discussion.

I slowly continued. "Of course, whenever a child has certain fractures that cannot be explained, you have to make sure that they weren't caused by someone else." On some strange level, it was a relief to say it.

She did not respond defensively. "I just can't believe this." The tearful mother looked off to one side toward the wall.

"I know this must be an awful shock," I tried to comfort, still unclear as to what role or knowledge, if any, the mother may have had concerning her daughter's injuries. She seemed convincing and genuinely concerned, speaking through her tears.

"I do appreciate your explaining all of this to me," she said. She would undoubtedly want explanations to many more questions, once the shock of the news wore off.

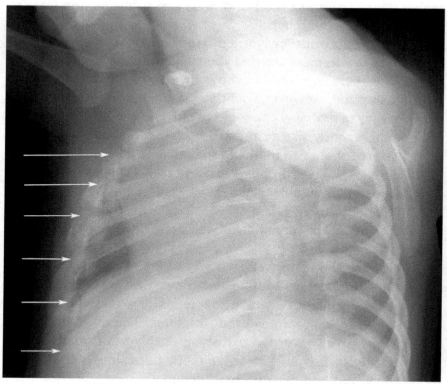

Rib fractures, non-accidental trauma (child abuse)
The baby girl's rib x-ray reveals healing fractures.

"I've already spoken with her pediatrician about the fractures, and he's waiting for you all to come back over to the office. He'll want to talk with you some more."

"Absolutely," she acknowledged through a few more tears. "We've just got to figure out who's *doing* this to her." She still sounded confused, understandably distraught, and a bit desperate. "Thank you."

"Not at all. Good luck to you, all of you, and I hope this all is resolved soon."

Either the mother was innocent and very concerned, or she was a really convincing actress. I did not know what to think and never met the other members of the family before they left the office.

I knew that the pediatrician was arranging a meeting with a social worker from the Child Protective Services Department. The family dynamics would be dissected and analyzed, in the hope of identifying the perpetrator and improving the circumstances that resulted in the physical abuse. I hoped and prayed that the baby would undergo no more inflicted injury. I also wondered whether the child would suffer any lasting physical or psychological damage from the trauma already experienced.

Had the child not had a cough that day, or had the pediatrician not ordered the film, the discovery of the injuries would have waited until later in the future, potentially after more injuries could have been inflicted. Perhaps the child might not have survived future trauma that might have occurred without the x-ray discoveries and the subsequent family investigation and intervention. Had I gotten so rushed in my work to miss seeing the rib fractures, the consequences could have been devastating.

The child's abuser obviously knows his or her own identity. Perhaps another person knows as well, but has not revealed the information. Regrettably, other people may never know, including the pediatrician and Protective Services Department staff. About two months passed, and I did not hear from the pediatrician. Finally, I called his office one day to report a different child's x-ray findings to him. I reminded him of the child whose fractures we had seen, and asked him whatever became of the investigation. All he knew was that neither parent was confirmed to be the guilty party. The parents had put the child in a different daycare facility, fearing that a daycare employee may have inflicted the injuries.

However, I never heard then of any local daycare facility or worker charged with physical abuse. When I looked up the child in our computer system years later when preparing this book, I found no further x-ray records for her. I am hoping that means that she needed no additional studies as she progressed from infancy to young adulthood. Maybe the family simply moved from the area.

In summary, whether the guilty party at the time was a member of the family, a daycare employee or babysitter, all evidence in this unresolved case suggests that the individual responsible for the abuse remained in a position of caring for children.

MIRROR IMAGE

The young woman had experienced upper abdominal pain for a couple of weeks. Her primary doctor found nothing on examination, prescribed some medication and antacids, and ordered an abdominal ultrasound to see if the patient might have gallstones.

No gallstones were found, but there was an issue: the ultrasound technologist could not find the woman's gallbladder at all, even though she had never had it removed. The gallbladder is a small sac typically just beneath the liver, in the upper right abdomen. Among its many functions, the liver makes bile, which helps us digest our food. Bile is excreted from the liver and stored in the gallbladder, until the time when someone consumes a meal. Eating triggers the gallbladder to contract its stored bile into the small intestine, aiding in digestion.

The technologist doing the ultrasound scan thought that the liver looked basically normal. It contained no mass or other abnormality like cirrhosis. However, the spleen in the upper left abdomen measured larger than average. An enlarged spleen can result from a variety of causes, ranging from liver disease to a viral infection or cancer. An abdominal CT scan was then recommended, to get a better picture of what was going on with her.

I met her the day of her CT scan. Greg, the tech doing the study, thought something looked awry, and asked me to check the images before he even got the patient off the scanner table.

The patient was in her thirties, pleasant, well dressed and articulate. Straightened jet-black bangs framed the forehead of her mahogany face. She looked comfortable and healthy.

"Hello," I introduced myself. "Greg here has asked me to look at your scan before you leave, if you can give us a few minutes."

"Of course. Take your time," she said. "I just hope everything is OK."

As soon as I began to scroll through the CT images on the scanner monitor, it became immediately evident that this was not going to be a normal scan. The organ in the upper left abdomen, where the spleen sits, was definitely larger than the average spleen. In contrast, in the upper right side was no ordinary looking liver. In fact, her right upper abdomen had not just one solid organ, but several similar-appearing organs grouped together, which had mimicked a normal liver on the ultrasound. Next to these, in the right upper abdomen, was the patient's stomach, which is normally on the left side.

On the opposite side of her diaphragm, the sheet of muscle separating the chest and abdomen, the woman's heart was on the normal left side. Below the diaphragm, however, everything was backward. Her pancreas extended to the right, not the normal left, and her intestines were opposite the normal position. She had a rare condition called situs inversus, where the abdominal organs are more or less in a mirror image, opposite-side location compared to most of us. For whatever reason, many patients with this condition also have more than one spleen, as did she. The collective spleens in her upper right abdomen had fooled the technologist doing her recent ultrasound into thinking that the patient had a normal sized liver in the usual location. That is, after all, what people expect to find. Sometimes, however, our assumptions are wrong, even when it comes to basic human anatomy.

Reading a scan where anatomy is rearranged—whether from surgery, or from embryological development, as in this case—generally takes longer than average. Our eyes and minds are accustomed to seeing organs in their expected locations. When structures are out of the usual place, the search pattern for disease takes longer. After more time reviewing—and temporarily inverting the images on the screen from right to left, so I could look at the organs the way I am used to seeing them—I ultimately decided that nothing else was wrong. No tumor, no infection or inflammation; and, a normal looking gallbladder, hidden deep in the upper left abdomen, where the ultrasound tech would have never thought to look for it.

"You've been in there for a while," she said guardedly, as Greg and I walked from the control room into the exam room, where she still lay on the scanner table.

"I didn't mean to make you worry," I apologized. "I just needed some time to look over your pictures, which are interesting. I read your paperwork as well, and understand that you started having abdominal pain a few weeks ago?"

"I did, but that's actually gone away," she explained. "My doctor thought it might just be acid irritating my stomach. I've been under a little stress lately at work. The pills he prescribed did seem to do the trick. But when they couldn't find my gallbladder, and said my spleen was enlarged, I wanted to keep the appointment for this test, even though I actually feel fine now. And I tested negative for hepatitis, which my doctor checked after learning that my spleen looked enlarged."

"That's good to know, and I'm glad you feel better. But I've got to ask, has anyone ever told you that you have any variations in your anatomy?"

She looked at me, puzzled. "No. What kind of variations do you mean?"

"Before the recent ultrasound, and this CT, I'm assuming you must have never had any kind of abdominal imaging test like these?"

"No, I had not," she said, looking more concerned.

"And you've never had surgery before in your abdomen?" I asked, understanding the answer to be *no* from her questionnaire.

"No, I've never had surgery of any kind."

"OK," I said, "let me explain what we're seeing. In most of us, the liver is up here," I gestured over my own abdomen, "in the right upper quadrant of the abdomen. The gallbladder is just below it, while the spleen and stomach are over on the upper left."

She nodded, seeming to have a basic understanding of human anatomy.

"Uncommonly, however, there are people whose internal organs are on the opposite sides. Some people just develop that way, when their organs are forming *in utero*. That looks to be the case with you. The reason they couldn't find your gallbladder is because they were looking in the wrong place in you. Yours is on the left, not the right. And what they thought was an enlarged spleen is actually a normal looking liver, just on the opposite side."

"Really?" she asked in half disbelief.

"Yes, it looks that way. And, what they thought was your liver is actually spleen tissue. Most people have just one spleen. But like other people with this condition, you actually have several spleens, grouped together, over on your right side."

"No one has ever told me this before," she said.

"If you never had any imaging done, I guess there's no reason you would have ever known it. Although have you at least had an x-ray done at some point? An x-ray of the abdomen, or the bottom part of a chest x-ray, might have at least shown your stomach on the right side instead of the left."

She thought. "I may have had an x-ray years ago, as a kid, but to be honest, I really don't remember. I've been pretty healthy, thank goodness."

"I think you still are healthy, just different on the inside. I need to look the pictures over more, but I didn't see anything actually wrong on the first glimpse, other than your organs being where they are."

She still looked puzzled, more confused than alarmed.

"It's a surprise," I said, "but better news than having anything actually wrong with your liver or spleen. Internal organs may reside where they usually do, but if you think about it: is there really an advantage to organs being on one side or the other? Or are they equally functional whether they form on the right or left, for whatever reason? We're not perfectly symmetric even on the outside, but definitely not on the inside. Having the liver and appendix on the right, the spleen and the lower colon on the left, are how most people are built. Being on the opposite side does not mean those organs don't work as well. It's just less common."

"How often do you see this?" she asked.

"It's rare, but not unheard of. I probably read over 10,000 cases a year, and off the top of my head, probably see this at least once or twice a year."

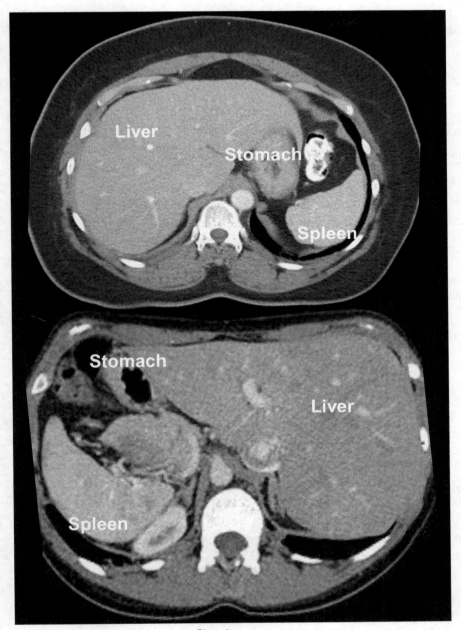

Situs inversus

Top image: Axial cross section of the upper abdomen with organs in their typical location.

Bottom image: Situs inversus. Axial image showing upper abdominal organs on the opposite sides typically seen.

She was not alarmed, but, with a perplexed expression, she asked the most basic of questions one can ask regarding her health: "Am I *normal?*"

I pondered her question. What could be more reassuring than to confirm that we are "normal," as most of us generally wish to be—however *normal* can be defined.

"Well, let's think about at it this way," I began to answer. "You are no longer in pain. You said you're typically healthy. I assume that includes having no physical limitations that you're aware of." She nodded.

I continued thinking aloud. "You've made it this far without even knowing that you were put together differently on the inside, because there's no effect. You feel fine, with no debilitation. So yes, you're normal; you're just *less average.*"

I did not say it, but that realization could even allow her to feel, perhaps, *special.*

"The fact is that most of us are walking around with some variation that we don't even know about. It might be a cyst, a benign growth, one kidney where there are usually two, or two arteries where there is usually one. We often just don't know these things until we go looking." She nodded in thought.

"That said," I countered, "I would recommend that you consider wearing one of those little medical bracelets, or at least carry in your wallet some kind of statement that you have this condition, called 'situs inversus, below the diaphragm.'" I wrote it down for her. "I say that only because, if you were ever in an accident or really sick, unable to communicate and possibly needing surgery, it would make things a whole lot easier for your doctors to know this in advance, rather than to have to discover it by surprise."

She understood. She thanked us and left the office, in her usual good condition. She required no additional medical tests before eventually moving out of town. I can only assume and hope that she is alive and well somewhere, still healthy, and still *normal*, despite being less average.

Pearls of Wisdom

S everal years into private practice and on my way toward partnership in the group, I was working an evening shift by myself at one of the hospitals our group staffed. Kathy, an ultrasound tech, brought me a case.

"Doctor, I'm going to need your help with this one," she began. "I've taken some pictures, but I'm not even sure if I'm looking at the right thing." She hung her films in front of me and we looked. If Kathy had not labeled in writing what part of the body she was scanning, I would not have known for sure by the images alone.

"What's the story here?" I asked. "This is a scrotal ultrasound?"

"Yes, on a one-month old boy who was born prematurely," she replied. "He had a scan a few weeks ago, which is here." She hung those films above the new ones to compare.

The infant had shown discoloration of his scrotal sac several days after his premature birth, and his doctor worried that the boy may have lost blood flow to his testicles. Each of the two testicles is suspended by a cord containing the arteries and veins that carry blood to and from the reproductive organs. If the cord twists, the blood flow can get cut off, and the testicle will die without emergency surgery to unravel the cord and restore blood flow. Making the diagnosis can be difficult, but is usually possible with ultrasound in older boys and grown men. Making the diagnosis in an infant is more difficult, because babies are unable to communicate where they hurt, and because the testicles are so small at that age and do not show much blood flow to begin with, even when healthy.

I looked at the old study from a few weeks back. That study was interpreted by a member of the group who was even younger and less experienced than I was, but his reading looked correct. The infant's testicles had been normal in size for his age, and the trace amount of blood flow seen on both sides then was within normal limits.

In the several weeks that had passed, the boy had gotten stronger and had finally left the hospital, to the great relief of his parents. He was eating well and gaining weight. However, his doctor had not been able to palpate the boy's testicles on a follow up office visit exam. The doctor wanted to take another look by ultrasound, even though the skin discoloration in that area had resolved.

"OK, let's see how it looks now," I said, shifting to the current study. What she had labeled as testicles looked different in size and shape than before. The labeled tissue definitely showed blood flow, in fact much more than before, and more than expected. The only problem was that I was not sure these were truly the testicles at all. Also filmed were a couple of pictures of something new in the upper scrotal sac on one side.

"You think these are the testicles?" I asked.

"I think so," she said in frustration, "but it was hard to get a good border, so I'm not sure about the measurements. Plus, he was moving most of the time."

"What did you think of this?" I asked, pointing to the newly seen small, round structure with a white periphery. "I've never seen anything quite like this before."

"I wasn't sure, I couldn't tell if it might be part of the cord in that location," she said. "This was a confusing scan."

"I see that. Let's go take a look together."

"Please," she encouraged.

We entered the dark ultrasound room, where I introduced myself to the parents. They were very pleasant, and shook my hand as the boy lay sleeping in his mother's lap.

"I hate to wake him, but let's lay him back down on the stretcher if we can and take another look," I said.

"Of course," they said while positioning the baby on the paper covered examination table. "How does everything look?" his father asked.

"I'm not sure yet. These scans can be a little tricky at this age," I replied.

The boy squirmed a bit, even though ultrasound scanning is painless. I tried to identify the testicles and thought I might have seen them where I expected to, but was not sure, because the distinction between testicle and adjacent thigh muscle was not that clear. Something else caught my eye: the small round structure with a white periphery seen high in the scrotum on one side had a matching, symmetric mate on the other side. Each was about the size of a small bean. I was not sure what they represented, but they just did not look right. They had not been on the images from the previous study, and they showed no blood flow as I scanned.

Often something symmetric on both sides of a child turns out to be a normal structure, typical for its stage of development. These, however, just did not seem normal. I was genuinely unsure, but wondered if they could be his testicles. If so, they no longer looked alive. I had seen testicles before that lost their blood supply, but never on both sides at the same time, nor in a child so young. The mere suggestion of such a diagnosis seemed awfully drastic.

"Let me tell you what we think so far," I tried to explain, simultaneously thinking aloud. "It's not easy to say, because we're trying to look at small structures to begin with, which don't show much blood flow anyway at this age." They listened attentively. "I'm also seeing something up high on both sides that looks a little different than in older males, not what we normally see, but the fact that they're symmetric makes me wonder if it might be normal." Wanting them to have some confidence in me and the technologist, I did not yet specify that neither Kathy nor I had seen anything quite like this before.

They rightfully looked a bit confused. "So what you're seeing looks normal?" the father asked.

"Possibly," I answered, but felt a pang of doubt. I wanted to be able to answer the question and make the call myself, but I did not feel confident in the assessment. I hated to admit it, but I did not know.

"Your son's scan is kind of a challenge to read," I confessed. "It does look a little different than it did a few weeks ago, when everything seemed OK. I'd like to show these pictures to a colleague and get a second opinion before we say for sure."

I feared their disapproval of my uncertainty, but they were completely understanding and appreciative of my desire to be more accurate. However, their response complicated the timing of the consult I was planning.

"That's fine," the mother said, "but the only thing is that we've got an appointment with the pediatric urologist tomorrow. We're supposed to take these films with us when we're done here."

Now the pressure was on. It would be easy enough to copy the films and show them to a colleague in the morning, but pride for myself, and for the quality and reputation of our practice, prevented me from sending out images with labeled notations that might be completely in error. I wanted to be right and did not want the urologist thinking we were idiots for not even being certain where the testicles were on the pictures.

"Let me go make a phone call and see if I can round up someone," I said, then left to track down the most senior pediatric radiologist in the group. He did not live that close to the hospital where I was working that evening, but he lived closer than the others I could ask. Images were still on film then, and remote access by internet was a bit cumbersome. If my more experienced colleague was going to assist, he would likely have to drive to the hospital. Fortunately, I caught him before he left the office where he was working that day. I explained the case, the unusual appearance of the findings, and the slight urgency for a formal reading.

"I hate to ask you this, Frank," I apologized as I explained the challenges of the case, "but do you think you might be able to take a look at this? I could have them try to send you the pictures at home to your computer if you prefer."

Without hesitation he came to the rescue. "Well, the problem with these is that you usually have to be there scanning live, as you know," he said in his slow, mildly southern drawl. "I'll swing by there on my way home. I'll try to be there in about forty-five minutes."

Relieved with the news of reinforcement, I reassured the parents that help was on the way if they could wait. They agreed without objection.

"This doctor is excellent," I described my colleague to them, "and is a specialist in pediatric radiology. He's got a lot more experience than I do." That was an understatement. Frank was sixty; I was still in my thirties. He had been reading x-rays since I was a child. He had trained before CT, ultrasound, and MRI were even available, and had learned to use these tools on the job and through educational courses, as the new technologies were introduced.

I had asked his opinions on several other children's x-rays during the preceding several years. Ironically, Frank had asked my opinion on a few occasions in helping to interpret CT and MRI scans. "You young folks have got the edge on us with your recent training," he would joke. "We old geezers are having trouble keeping up."

Rush hour traffic was bad, and the parents patiently waited over an hour until the tall, spectacled, silver-haired specialist arrived at the hospital. I showed him the pictures privately, and pointed out the symmetric, small round structures with the white peripheries.

"Surely these aren't his testicles, are they? If they are, they're smaller than they were before, and no longer show blood flow. I've never seen them look quite like this. You'd wonder if they had scarred or even partially calcified on the surface, with that bright border. That can't be good." On one level, I knew that these findings might imply that both of the small glands had already lost their blood supply, but I just did not want to believe that.

Frank looked at the images. He said nothing, but wheels were turning inside his brain while his face revealed that he was rapt in thought.

We then went to the examining room. With a calmness and reassurance that immediately put the parents at ease, he introduced himself and asked a few questions, then began scanning for a few minutes. This time the baby slept. Without the baby's motion from earlier, the images were sharper and borders easier to delineate. What the ultrasound tech and I had initially wanted to believe might be normal testicles, with above average blood flow, now clearly looked like normal nearby groin muscle tissue, not testicles. Frank then focused on the small bean-sized structures, confirmed the absence of blood flow, and took some measurements.

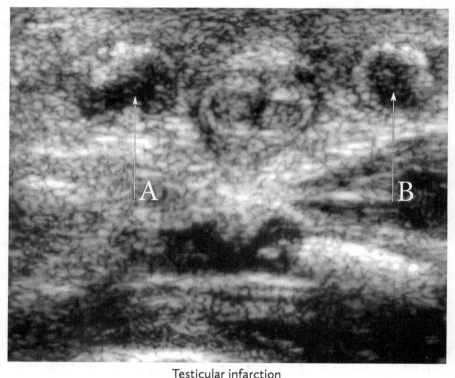

Testicular infarction
The labeled small oval-shaped structures (A) and (B) with bright periphery represent the baby boy's testes which had lost their blood supply.

I feared, in fact knew on one level, that we were confirming the diagnosis I had never seen before quite like this, and I had dared not make the call without his backup.

"Those are the testicles," he confirmed. They had looked all right on the prior ultrasound a few weeks before, when the scrotal skin had been discolored, but at the microscopic level they probably had already lost their blood supply and been damaged back then. I do not know if anything could have been done a few weeks beforehand, given the difficulty in making the diagnosis at that time, but it was certainly too late to save them now.

He took over the discussion with the parents, pausing while choosing his words carefully. I stood back and listened, no longer the voice of authority, grateful for his reinforcement.

"These kinds of cases can be tough," he began, "and I can see why Dr. Ruff here wanted to run this by someone."

"We sure appreciate your coming in," the boy's mother said as her husband nodded in agreement. I appreciated it even more.

"What do you think is going on?" the husband asked. The couple was still gracious, but normal parental concern was showing through.

"Well, after taking a look myself, I am afraid that his testicles may have indeed lost their blood supply. The fact that they've gotten smaller, and that their appearance has changed, are worrisome findings."

"What does this mean?" the mother asked. The father stared at Frank, awaiting a response.

"In terms of his actual development, less than you might fear," he consoled. "Doctors have gotten very good at being able to administer hormones when the time comes. So with regard to his growing and going through puberty, he can develop normally and live a normal life in that regard."

"But does this mean he won't be able to have children?" the mother asked, still composed outwardly, but sounding more surprised and guarded.

"I wasn't going to burden you with that just yet," he hesitated, "but since you've asked specifically—if we're right about his diagnosis, then no, he would not be able to."

A brief but painful moment slowly passed in silence.

"But he would be OK himself, with regard to his own health?" the father asked. His wife now stared at the doctor and said nothing.

"His own growth and development should be normal with treatments," Frank reiterated. "Again, I'm sorry to lay so much on you at one time. I know this is not the news any parent wants to hear, but I'm not going to lie to you, since you did ask."

"No, we wouldn't want that," the father said.

"No," said the mother, "we appreciate you being honest, even though it's sure not what we were hoping to hear."

We gave them a set of the ultrasound films that Frank had acquired. I discarded the earlier films that Kathy and I had taken. We wished the family luck, and they drove home in the dark.

"I can't believe it," I told Frank. "I'm so glad you came in. I've seen testicular torsion on one side before, but never an infant with a bilateral infarction like this."

"It's not common, fortunately, but premature infants are the ones who can get it." He shook his head. "I hated having to tell them that information, that mother in particular; but since she specifically asked, I just couldn't dodge the question."

"No, you couldn't," I agreed. "At least you knew about the hormone therapy. That should help soften the blow."

He shook his head. "Maybe. I still hate being the bearer of bad news."

"We all do. I also hate not knowing what I'm looking at. But sometimes you genuinely just don't know. Other times you do have an idea, but you don't want to believe it. You'd like to make it turn out better if you could."

"I know," he said.

"I can't thank you enough for coming to my rescue," I said. "Please apologize to your wife for me for your late arrival home."

"Oh, she's pretty understanding," he smiled. "I hope the rest of your evening goes more smoothly."

"Thanks."

He turned and headed for the door. As he approached the exit, I called to him.

"Frank, if you're still wondering whether or not you all in the more senior category are providing valuable input, please rest assured and wonder no more."

"I appreciate that," he smiled.

(Note: On a follow up ultrasound a few weeks later, the testes had completely atrophied and disappeared, with no residual tissue visible.

The child apparently had a perfectly healthy boyhood, enjoying school and sports like the rest of his peers, and is normal in height. Hormone treatments began when he hit his teenage years, and he is reportedly doing fine as well at this stage of development.)

Surprise

One October afternoon, a twenty-nine year-old woman weighing over 300 pounds came in for the first ultrasound of her first pregnancy. The young woman was escorted by her boyfriend, who was quick to point out that his girlfriend would soon be his legal wife. The couple sheepishly revealed that their pregnancy was unplanned and only recently discovered. For several years she had been taking hormone injections every few months as a means of birth control, and had no menstrual period for those few years while she had been receiving the injections. Because she had no periods, she had no idea that she had also missed a few for a very different reason. Only upon visiting a doctor that week for recent leg swelling did she have a medical work up which included a pregnancy test.

The doctor who diagnosed the woman's pregnancy attempted to do a manual pelvic examination, but it was of limited value, given the patient's size. Estimating the gestation at approximately three months, she ordered an ultrasound to date the pregnancy more accurately.

Rick, the ultrasound technologist, began the study, scanning and trying to take pictures of the moving baby. He immediately observed that this baby was way beyond three months in development. Before trying to take pictures of organs typically studied during pregnancy, like the spine, heart, kidneys, and brain, he first obtained measurements of the skull, abdominal circumference, and femur length in order to estimate the baby's gestational age.

Those measurements he could obtain, but studying the baby's anatomy was more challenging. Ultrasound waves typically have a hard time penetrating through more tissue, so detail is usually clearer in a smaller mother than a larger one. Some organs like brain are also easier to see before the skull develops further, with more calcium deposited in the bone, blocking ultrasound waves. The unexpectedly advanced age of the fetus compounded the study's limitations. While Rick did his best to obtain measurements and take pictures, the couple began asking questions.

"We have no idea how long she's been pregnant," the fiancé said, "because she hasn't had a real period in several years on account of the shots."

"The doctor thought I was about three months on my exam," she said. "How does it look so far?"

Rick answered, reserving the details for me. "You're way farther along than three months."

"How much farther?" she asked.

"You're in your third trimester."

"You mean I've got less than three months to go?!" she exclaimed, astonished. Her fiancé looked stunned.

"Less than that, in fact. I need to check these measurements with our charts and show the pictures to the doctor, who will come in to talk with you in a minute."

"Do you see anything wrong?" she asked worriedly. The father-to-be sat perplexed in silence.

"No, I haven't seen anything abnormal, although we can't see everything in a baby this far along. Let me show these to the doctor and we'll be back soon."

A few minutes later he brought me the images and measurements to review. "You're not going to believe this."

A standard term pregnancy, dating from a woman's last menstrual period before conception until the day of delivery, averages about forty weeks. The ultrasound he had performed demonstrated a single living fetus, with an age estimate of thirty-eight weeks. Due in only two weeks, this pregnancy was essentially term. She could deliver any day now.

"She didn't know she was pregnant at all?" I quizzed him in disbelief. "You've got to be kidding. How could she not know? Despite her lack of menstrual cycles, didn't she feel pain, movement, nausea, *something*? Good thing she didn't go into early labor, or they would have really had a surprise."

By the time we entered the room, the expectant mother was in such shock that she was nearly unable to speak for several minutes. She was still lying on the table, staring at the ceiling, with her hands covering her mouth. She was indeed a big woman, so large that I could not tell she was pregnant until I scanned her myself.

The boyfriend shook his head in wide-eyed disbelief, but did his best to reassure his fiancée. "Don't worry. It'll be all right. Everything will be fine, honey," he said, comforting himself as much as her.

Once she regained some composure, she spoke. "Oh, my God. I don't know where to begin. OK, tell me, when exactly is the due date? No—don't tell me, write it down first, please."

The request was a bit unusual, since they were going to read it immediately anyway, but the technologist simply looked ahead two weeks on the calendar, wrote the due date down on a piece of paper, and handed it to the couple.

"Oh! Oh my God!" she exclaimed, while her fiancé shook his head again in reaction to the unexpected news that had still not sunk in yet. They needed a few additional moments before resuming the conversation.

A professional and personal curiosity overcame me. "I know this is your first pregnancy, but you truly had no symptoms that made you think you might be pregnant? You haven't felt any movement or had any pain?"

She exhaled slowly. "About a month ago I was having some discomfort and rumbling in my stomach, but it went away, and I thought it was just gas pains. The birth control shots worked fine for so long that it never bothered me that I quit having periods. How am I going to explain this to my *family*?"

"If you can deal with the news, so can they," I tried to reassure. "Just once more, other than that, you don't remember having any nausea early on? Unusual food cravings? Any changes in your skin, your sleep, anything?"

"No," she replied, almost in a whisper, then finally shifted her gaze from the ceiling to concentrate on our faces. "I know you're supposed to take vitamins when you're pregnant. Because I didn't know, I wasn't doing that on a regular basis."

"What we can see on the ultrasound, including the baby's spine, looks normal, as best as we can tell."

Her fiancé interjected. "We were talking before you came into the room. She's worried about some prescription painkillers she's had to take at times for her back."

"That's not all," she confessed. "I'm not a daily drinker at all, but there were a few times several months ago when I had a few drinks on occasion, going out with some friends. I had no idea I was pregnant! Have I harmed the baby?"

I tried to soothe their concern. "Here's the way I look at it. We can't see everything by ultrasound on a baby this far along, but what we see on your study today looks normal. Also, remember that a lot of our mothers a generation or two ago drank, smoked, or took medications with less knowledge of it affecting us, and most of us turned out fine. The odds are that everything is normal."

The couple seemed somewhat relieved, but they were still recovering from the shock of the news.

"That's all I can tell you regarding the ultrasound," I concluded. "Let me go call your doctor and let her know what we see. Be sure to follow up with her today in order to make some plans. You've also got a few things you may want to take care of, like getting some baby supplies, including a car seat."

"Oh, we've got a *lot* to do," her fiancé confirmed.

"This is just so unreal," she continued. "I'm going to be so embarrassed to tell my mother and the rest of the family, and everybody at work. I guess I'll be taking some time off. Has this ever happened to you before? Have you ever seen this?"

"In my personal experience, no. When I was a medical student on the OB/GYN rotation, I saw one teenage girl who delivered a term infant at home, and then she was brought to the hospital. She was small, yet swore to me that neither she nor her family suspected that she had been pregnant. She even claimed that her clothes still fit her. Only when I quizzed her further did she reluctantly admit that she kind of wondered. I think she was just the biggest case of denial I've ever seen."

They nodded without uttering a word.

"However," I continued, "a couple of colleagues of mine have seen this happen, including seeing women come to the ER with unexplained abdominal and pelvic pain, who are then discovered to be in active labor. I wouldn't call it common, but cases like yours are far from isolated." I paused, but figured she was beyond being offended in her state of near shock. "Of course, they're usually not size-two women."

"No, I understand that," she admitted.

"Well, thank God we found out when we did, right baby?" the boyfriend tried to comfort.

"Honey, please call me anything but *baby* today," she tried to joke, although neither laughed.

I wished them well and sent them on their way, reminding them that I would call her doctor immediately. The family practitioner who had examined the patient was as shocked as the couple themselves, but grateful for the information while the baby was at least still *in utero*. We were all struck by how drastically and permanently the couple's lives had changed with one ultrasound study, with more dramatic changes ahead only a couple of weeks later.

SPARED

The phone rang at the beginning of the work day, on what had begun as a routine Tuesday morning at the hospital. "You've got an abscess drainage today in CT on a ten year-old girl," my colleague explained to me over the telephone. "I got consent from the mom late yesterday. We couldn't do the procedure without anesthesia, and they were busy in other cases. One of the parents should be in later this morning, but again, I already got consent. The little girl had surgery for ruptured appendicitis about ten days ago, and now she's got a couple of abscesses big enough to drain. They know this may not be enough. She still might need another operation, but the surgeons want to try this first."

The CT pictures showed just what he described: several infected fluid collections in her abdominal cavity, two of which were large enough for me to remove by inserting plastic drains.

I walked out of the dark reading room into the fluorescent lighted CT scan control area, witnessing activity through the windows of each of the adjoining scanner rooms. Technologists were moving patients on and off the CT tables, hooking up mechanical fluid injectors to the IVs in patients' arms. Transporters were bringing patients to and from the department by wheelchair or stretcher. Trauma surgery residents crowded around one scanner while their patient from an auto collision got scanned. Telephones were ringing, from nurses wanting to know when their patients would be imaged, to doctors adding on cases.

"What time is anesthesia going to be ready to do the drainage on the girl?" I asked the lead tech at the phone desk.

"This morning—soon. I just called for her to come down."

Another tech, a young woman with short hair and a stout

frame, burst into the room from the corridor. "They said on the news just now that a plane hit the World Trade Center."

"Really?" we asked. "How? What happened?"

"I don't know yet, they just started reporting it. But it wasn't a small plane, it was a big commercial jet."

After what seemed like only a few minutes, the same tech went out to check on the news, then resurfaced, flustered and distraught. "Now the second tower was also hit by a plane. It's a terrorist attack. The planes were hijacked."

While people in the department did not abandon their jobs, they did tune in to broadcasts on the radios available, and they tried to continue working. Periodically people also stepped out to the waiting room to watch TV news footage. Two colleagues even thought of a much less conventional way to obtain news then: they logged onto the internet. Various coworkers took unofficial turns announcing updates aloud to everybody within earshot in the department. Much of the information turned out to be erroneous, but confirming anything at the moment was next to impossible, given all the turmoil and confusion.

The worry was palpable, the shock hard to comprehend. In the waiting area, family members bringing in patients for studies stood next to hospital employees wearing green scrubs and white coats, everyone fixated on the televised news reports. Some people began to cry. Yet despite the distraction and concern, we still had patients to take care of, and could not abandon our primary duties.

Tension was mounting, but we tried to control our distraction— until the same CT tech who had announced the planes hitting the World Trade Center entered our work area once more in a frenzy, visibly upset, her voice loud and slightly unsteady. "Now a plane has hit the Pentagon," she blurted out. "We're under attack."

"*The Pentagon?* How could a plane hit the Pentagon?! I would have thought it would be the best defended building in the world!"

"They said it was a big explosion. A lot of people may have died."

"And those that didn't...I wonder if any will be brought here. We're one of the closest major trauma centers." Fear mounted on everyone's faces.

The lead tech got my attention. "The girl for the abscess drainage is here."

Preoccupied with the shocking news, and mentally preparing for a potential shipment of casualties from the nearby Pentagon, it took effort to concentrate on the one patient I could actually help at the moment. I had to focus.

The anesthesiologist was setting up for sedation in the CT scan room, and the nurse who had come down with the girl introduced me to our young blue-eyed patient. "This is Amanda," the friendly nurse smiled. "I understand her mom gave consent already. She spent the night with Amanda but just left, because Amanda's got some young siblings at home," she explained, "but her dad may be coming in later."

For a sick kid in the hospital, receiving IV antibiotics and about to undergo a minor procedure, Amanda looked remarkably under control.

"You're going to be fine," I tried to reassure her, and she smiled just slightly. "With the medicines this other doctor gives you, you'll be asleep and shouldn't feel a thing. And when we've gotten that infected fluid out of there, you should be feeling better tomorrow than you do today."

The anesthesiologist gave her a deep sedative, and we proceeded with her procedure, a respite from the distractions of the horrific national news. Amanda's drainage tube placements went smoothly. Only after the case was finished did techs, nurses, and other doctors fill me in on the latest news updates, and the many unsubstantiated rumors, circulating in a whirlwind.

Several of us tried to call local loved ones but could not get through on the telephone. A surgeon on duty then walked through the CT department, confirming that we still might be receiving some casualties from the Pentagon site, and she wanted to discuss how best to expedite scanning the neediest trauma patients. However, we ended up not receiving any victims to my knowledge. Most of the casualties were mortal.

"Her father's here now, in the hall outside," the CT tech informed me. I stepped out to meet him. He had a short haircut and a trim, solid build. His outward strength was further complemented by his polite manner and patience. He wore civilian clothes, but when I later learned that he was a military officer, that came as no surprise. The rest of the story, however, was a surprise I shall never forget.

"She did great," I said. "She was brave and very cooperative. It went just fine."

"I'm glad to hear it. They said she still might need a second operation, but we'd love to avoid that if we could. Thanks for all your help."

"You're more than welcome. I do hope it works. At the very least, her pain and fevers should improve after getting that pus out of there. Chances are pretty good that she can avoid a second operation."

Relieved, he gave me a thumbs up.

"Good luck with her recovery," I said, extending my right arm.

"Thanks again," he said, shaking my hand.

I turned and started to walk down the hall, but for some reason, perhaps an innate impulse to connect to someone else's humanity that memorable morning, I stopped after only a few steps. Turning back, I voiced the obvious thought on my mind. "I might as well tell you that I'll never forget her procedure, given the events of today."

"Tell me about it," he said, with unimaginable composure. "I work at the Pentagon—in the section they say got hit this morning. I'm worried about the people I work with. I've tried to call but haven't been able to get through on the phone. The only reason I'm not at work today is because I knew you were going to do this procedure on my daughter, and I wanted to be here for her sake."

SECTION IV:
FOREIGN BODIES

Inanimate objects, often man-made, can find their way into people—sometimes for good reason, often times not. Implanted medical devices certainly abound, including surgical clips and staples, pacemakers and defibrillators, vascular stents, shunts, artificial heart valves, joint replacements, fracture fixation hardware, insulin pumps, nerve stimulators, hernia mesh, tubal ligation clips or wires, intrauterine devices and penile implants. Each surgical device tells a story of a condition or status, illness or injury, and an attempted repair or adjustment.

Then there are the nonmedical objects. Soldiers, crime victims, and other unlucky individuals may have retained bullets or shrapnel. Other accident victims may have metal, glass, even gravel or wood fragments embedded in their bodies, with any number of complications resulting. I have seen many a patient who has accidentally swallowed a fish bone, which can sometimes get caught in the throat, requiring extraction. In one patient, a fish bone punctured the intestinal wall, also requiring surgery. In other incidents, patients have inadvertently swallowed metal wires that had broken off barbecue grill brushes, the wires lodging in the tongue base or throat and requiring surgical extraction.

Foreign objects are sometimes introduced on purpose. Some disturbed youth occasionally insert metal objects under their skin—not the myriad piercings we all now see, but objects like pins, metal wires, or paper clips. These can cause infections, among other complications, and are sometimes inadvertently discovered when x-rays are obtained for accidents or other reasons. Foreign bodies may also be intentionally ingested. People with varying degrees of mental illness have been known to swallow all sorts of objects—batteries, pebbles, safety pins, thumb tacks, even broken glass. On one occasion I saw a patient who had swallowed a razor blade, and remarkably, it passed without surgical intervention.

Metallic tattoos can also be visible under x-ray. The most memorable such tattoo to pass my computer screen thus far was that of a 350-pound woman having a CT scan. On her abdomen, in neatly embedded metallic beads, was the word **SEXY**.

Small children may inhale peanuts, or swallow coins. Super strong small batteries were featured in news stories a few years ago, after some children swallowed more than one magnet. The magnets were so strongly attracted to each other that they fixed two adjacent bowel loops together, causing obstructions that required surgery.

Most radiologists have also seen more than a few foreign bodies trapped down below, objects that were used for sexual pleasure. In women, I have seen a light bulb lodged, globe end first. And worse, a glass soft drink bottle in a different young woman who did not even know it was there. She had had a wild weekend in a motel room with a couple of less than gentle men, and did not remember the details of their time together, due to the drugs involved. When she came to the hospital a couple of days later, complaining of pelvic pain, an x-ray revealed the bottle.

In men, I have seen even more such scenarios, and the spectrum of patients has ranged from young and single, to older and in long-term heterosexual marriages. Lodged sex toys, a cucumber, and a zucchini for starters, as well as a shower head that broke off from the portable spray nozzle and could not pass on its own. One unfortunate man got excessively rough with a plunger handle, causing a small tear in his colon that fortunately healed without surgery, but did require drainage of an abscess, plus IV antibiotics. A completely nonjudgmental word of caution: I'm all for people enjoying their lives and the pleasure zones our bodies provide, but please be careful. Don't hurt yourself or others; and make sure that there is some sort of strap or foolproof handle on anything that may go in, to make sure that it can come out safely and easily at home.

Enough of the graphic or salacious.

Like other parts of this collection, the stories selected for this section date from internship, through training, and into practice. The foreign bodies, the patients, and the circumstances are all different. They shed light on what may be going on in people's lives, the challenges that some have to overcome, and the extreme circumstances in which people sometimes find themselves. They may force us to reexamine our vulnerability, and, in at least two stories, they examine the limitations of health care, or of medical knowledge in general, despite the best of intentions.

CRYING WOLF

The woman was only in her late sixties, but she seemed more than a decade older. She had been assigned to me in the medical clinic during my internship. Unlike most of the kind and gracious elderly ladies in that southeastern coastal town, this woman was typically grouchy, like a bitter pill in a sea of sweet tea. Her face was sallow, her eyebrows furrowed, and she wore a nearly perpetual scowl. When we first met during her clinic appointment, she immediately began listing her symptoms, insistent and urgent that I get a full picture of her physical woes.

She had a number of common chronic ailments, including diabetes, high blood pressure, and a hypoactive thyroid gland, but these conditions were reasonably controlled with medications. A former smoker, she did suffer from emphysema, a weak heart, and peripheral arterial disease, limiting the blood flow through her narrowed vessels. She could not walk very far without assistance and was often tired. She also complained of numerous aches and pains throughout her body, from deep inside to her extremities. Nevertheless, treating her was usually a matter of titrating long-term medications, encouraging healthy activities, and verbal reassurance, as there rarely seemed to be anything acutely wrong with her, despite her complaints and chronic conditions.

She was widowed, but volunteered no details about her former husband. I do not recall if she had any grown children, but I distinctly remember that no relative ever accompanied her during her visits to the clinic or emergency room.

Although I never told her so, I did pity the woman, for a combination of reasons. She was fairly decrepit, particularly for her age, and she had no visible family support. She was also financially indigent. But with all of those problems, her negative outlook was also a concern. The sick are as entitled to feel the way they do as anyone else, but I had known so many other people who dealt with illness and life's other challenges more positively or hopefully than she did, and who ended up living more rewarding lives as a result. It may be easy for others to say, particularly a healthy outsider, but I could not help but think that an attitude adjustment might give her a perspective that could make her feel better in body and spirit, both areas where she was sorely in need.

Medicaid and Medicare paid some of her bills, enabling her to live at a nearby assisted living facility, where she was determined to stay. Despite her unsolicited and freely expressed dislike of the place, she dreaded even more the thought of ending up in a nursing home. That streak of determination in her demeanor was admirable, and it gave me hope that she might still try to be proactive in maintaining her diminished but residual health and independence, rather than give up altogether.

Unlike other patients who were at least partially resigned to the effects of time, this woman was bitter that she did not feel as well as she wished. She openly vocalized her dissatisfaction with her condition, often requesting mild prescription narcotics "to ease her uncontrollable pain." She had been assigned to other medical residents, during the years before my internship, and had received a fairly extensive evaluation for her varying complaints. An abdominal ultrasound had shown no gallstones. Knee x-rays revealed only mild arthritis. Atherosclerosis affected her blood vessels, but not bad enough to require bypass surgery. Blood tests indicated appropriate control of her diabetes and thyroid condition. Breathing treatments kept her emphysema steady. The tests ordered at various times may have changed, but her ailments and attitude did not. We may have been missing something in her workup, but I could not figure out what it might be.

Whenever I saw her, her opening statement remained consistently negative, and slightly demanding. She expressed discontent with her doctors and nurses, angry that we could not do more to boost her low energy level and abate her vague diffuse pains. She was often critical and consistently unpleasant. I never recall her expressing any thanks to those trying to help her. She was the opposite of endearing, and, frankly, I did not look forward to seeing her.

One Sunday morning I was assigned to help staff the hospital emergency room. Bright and early at 7 a.m., an ambulance arrived, and the paramedics wheeled this woman in from the parking lot. She was sitting up on her stretcher, though leaning to one side, with the usual scowl on her face. The ambulance driver had not bothered to use the siren or flashing lights, as the patient was in no particular distress. Nevertheless, her assisted living staff had asked that she be taken to the emergency room for evaluation of her worsening weakness. We ran the battery of usual tests and found no acute problem. Blood and urine tests were negative, her EKG was stable, and her chest x-ray down the hall was read as having nothing acute since prior studies. Determining that she was not sick enough for hospital admission, I called the woman's assisted living facility to let them know that she would be returning. The facility director answered the phone.

"Good morning," I began, "I'm calling to give you the discharge information on one of your residents sent here for evaluation this morning."

"No," he interrupted. "She *was* a resident. She has been sent to the hospital and has lost her room here."

"I know she's here now," I said, "but we are releasing her back to you. We evaluated her here in the emergency room and cannot find any reason to admit her."

He paused briefly, but his irritation increased. "She can't come back here," he insisted. "She didn't work out here, and has lost her room."

I was briefly confused, then temporarily speechless. I was just an intern a few months out of medical school, but I knew the facility director was acting not only unprofessionally, but also possibly illegally.

"Sir, there is no way that you have vacated her belongings and moved another resident into that room during the past three hours, on a Sunday morning no less. We find no reason to admit this woman to the hospital today. You cannot kick her out just because you have called an ambulance to send her to the emergency room. She will be returning shortly by that same ambulance, and I will see her in my clinic next week."

When I did see her the following week, she was feeling strong enough to provide her usual list of mild, chronic complaints, but agreed that she was a little better. Satisfied with her improvement, I sent her on her way.

A couple of months later, she returned for another clinic visit. A medical student was shadowing me that day, and I briefed her outside of the examination room door.

"This one can be a challenge," I told the student. "She's a bit of a malcontent." We opened the door and entered the room.

"Hello, ma'am, how are you feeling today?" I asked.

"I'm not doing a bit of good," she replied. "I hurt all over, just awful." Her temperature and blood pressure were normal. Her hands slightly trembled. She seemed more agitated than usual, but it was unclear why. I even wondered if she might be overacting for the medical student, whom she had not previously met.

"Let's take a listen to your heart and lungs," I said. The student and I pulled out our stethoscopes. The woman's pulse was normal, her heart rhythm regular. However, one of her lung bases sounded abnormal, with crackling sounds during deep inspiration.

"How has your breathing been?" I asked.

"Terrible as usual," she said. "I've been using my inhalers, but it just doesn't get any better."

"Have you been coughing?" the student asked.

"I cough all the time," she replied. "That never goes away."

"Are you getting anything up when you cough?" she asked pertinently.

"I always have a little phlegm," she said. "I've been suffering that for years. You all have got to do something, because I just don't feel good, period."

I still was not convinced that she had anything newly wrong with her, wondering if her abnormal breath sounds might be from her emphysema. The rest of her examination was unremarkable. Perhaps she came in to the clinic because she was lonely, a social outcast at the rest home, and wanted some attention or reassurance.

"We'll be right back," we said as we briefly exited the room to talk in the hallway.

"What did you think?" I asked the student.

"I'm not sure. She's obviously kind of debilitated for someone her age. She doesn't have a fever, or any change in her chronic cough, but her lungs sounded abnormal," she said. "I was wondering if she might have a pneumonia, or maybe a little congestive heart failure?"

"She doesn't have any leg swelling, and has never had congestive failure to my knowledge. It could just be from her emphysema."

"Maybe," she said, pensively, while perhaps trying not to offend my minimal level of greater experience than hers. "Has she sounded like that before?"

"I'm not sure," I admitted, "not that I remember. But she has had a lot of work up over the years. She is obviously not in great shape, but she always says that something is bothering her. We seldom find anything new. I hate to order tests unnecessarily."

"I know," she countered, "but, if her lungs may sound different, I would have probably gotten the x-ray."

"I guess you're right," I reluctantly acknowledged, shamed by my student who turned out to be my teacher that day. "One chest x-ray wouldn't be unreasonable."

While I was seeing another patient, the radiologist called and informed the clinic nurse that the old woman had pneumonia, new since her last chest x-ray. Busy with other patients in the clinic, I quickly wrote a prescription for some antibiotics, hoping that she would improve from the pills and not require hospitalization. She seemed stable enough to be treated as an outpatient, and would be observed by her rest home staff in case she got worse. I also knew that, if we did put her in the hospital, she truly would lose her rest home bed, with the unscrupulous administrator doing everything in his power to find a nicer and possibly wealthier replacement.

After the last patient was seen that day, the last prescription written, and the last clinic visit note dictated, I proceeded to the radiology department to see the woman's chest x-ray film. Only months away from beginning my radiology residency training, I was eager to see my patients' x-rays and not just read the reports, particularly when the studies were abnormal. Her films revealed the pneumonia, plus signs of emphysema. The films also revealed something I had not known about the patient: she had multiple pieces of shotgun pellets scattered over half of her chest. Review of older chest x-rays in her jacket showed that the pellets had been there a long time. Because the shooting was old, many of the recent chest x-ray reports had not even mentioned it. The woman's skin had also healed with no visible scars. Nevertheless, someone had once fired a shotgun at her years ago, leaving metallic pieces in her body for the rest of her life, buried beneath her skin but immortalized on her x-ray film.

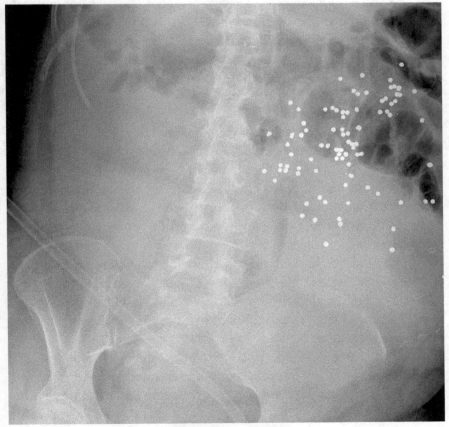

Shotgun pellets
The small white objects are metallic pellets embedded in a patient who was previously shot.

Evidently the hospital and rest home staff were not the only people who had ever found this woman to be disagreeable or unpleasant. Either she was once simply in the wrong place at the wrong time, or someone in her past had taken a much stronger disliking to her, attempting to remove her from the ranks of the living human population.

The woman returned two weeks later for a follow-up clinic visit, to assess her progress after the antibiotic treatment. It was the first time that I noticed her actually revealing a touch of some satisfaction. She clearly looked better than on her previous visits, and she reluctantly acknowledged that she did indeed feel improved after the antibiotics. She was rather quick to point out that she still would like more energy, and that she was not in nearly as good a shape as she used to be. Nevertheless, she showed a hint of a smile beneath her perpetual but softened scowl. She blushed when I complimented her on her improved appearance, with the corners of her lips slightly turning upward.

I listened to her lungs, and confirmed that the abnormal breath sounds had cleared.

"I want to send you for another x-ray, just to make sure that the film shows no more pneumonia." The thought triggered my recollection of her previous chest film. "There is one other thing I wanted to ask you about. I couldn't help but notice on your x-ray a couple of weeks ago that you have been shot in the past. Your previous doctors must have known that, but you never mentioned it to me before."

The woman looked down, then looked away to the side, and lost what little smile she had briefly displayed. She folded her hands, her fingers slightly trembling. "Well, there are some things that I just may not want to talk about," she replied, never glancing up to meet my gaze.

On hearing that one pertinent but indelicate question, she reverted from slightly improved and encouraged back to dejected, pained, and pitiful. The details of her shooting could have provided insight into her domestic history, and may have been more medically relevant, depending on the extent of the injuries. That information would never be forthcoming however, and my ability to help her would remain limited. Her physical body was indeed not as strong as it had once been, and now her briefly improved spirits were quickly beaten down by my inquiry into an incident she would rather, but could never, forget.

"That's okay," I tried to console. "You keep up the good work. It's good to see you feeling better."

System Failure

The woman had undergone a hysterectomy several days beforehand, necessitated by benign uterine fibroid tumors that caused heavy bleeding. She was over forty, desired no more children, and looked forward to a more simplified life without the monthly symptoms she had endured for several years.

After the operation, her recovery in the hospital progressed slower than expected. She had a bit more pain than most women experience. The obstetrics and gynecology residents taking care of her ordered an abdominal x-ray to evaluate her abdominal pain, but the film helped very little. The patient moved during the x-ray exposure, and the film cassette was not centered properly by the x-ray student taking the bedside film. The lower half of the patient's abdomen was excluded from view. The radiologist reading the film called it non-diagnostic and recommended that it be repeated. However, no repeat film was performed by the student, or the x-ray tech supervising, and the gynecologists taking care of the patient did not order a repeat study.

The woman remained in the hospital several more days after her hysterectomy. Her pain was relatively mild, but it persisted. The OB/GYN residents taking care of her then ordered a pelvic ultrasound, which I read with my professor. Only a small abnormality was revealed that day.

I called the gynecology resident to discuss the findings. "As you might imagine," I began, "an ultrasound this soon after surgery is a bit limited. We can only press so hard near her incision, and she's got a lot of bowel gas blocking our view." The woman's painkillers likely made that problem worse, as narcotics impair the normal motion of intestinal smooth muscle, causing gas distension and constipation.

"Her ovaries look OK, with normal blood flow, but we do see some fluid in the left side of her pelvis. It's a small collection, but it looks complex. Is there any chance she has an infection?" I asked.

"We don't think so," she replied. "She has no fever or white count."

"Well, it could always be a little post-op hemorrhage," I said. "The problem is that we can't tell the difference by ultrasound between blood and pus."

"Yeah, I know," she said. "Her ovaries looked good at the time of surgery. Anything else?"

"That's all we can see today. Of course any time we see a complex fluid collection, we recommend that she have a repeat ultrasound within a couple of months, unless she develops other symptoms and needs a workup sooner," I advised.

"We'll see how she does," she responded.

Odds were most likely that the small fluid collection was simply some normal hemorrhage post recent surgery. The resident did not order a follow-up ultrasound during the suggested time interval.

Five months later, the woman returned to the gynecology clinic, complaining of gradually worsening pain ever since her surgery. Her dark hair was pulled back, revealing faint black circles beneath her eyes and a face drained of energy.

"I know other women who have had hysterectomies, and most tell me that they felt back to normal after a couple of months," she sighed with visible fatigue. "I've been patient since my surgery, but I thought I would be doing better than this by now. I've even started having low-grade fevers. I'm getting really tired of not feeling well for so long." She had undergone the hysterectomy to have an improved quality of life, but she had yet to experience the anticipated benefit.

The clinic doctor ordered another pelvic ultrasound, which showed that the complex fluid collection in her left pelvis had grown since the ultrasound right after surgery five months earlier. In addition to the larger size, the fluid collection now demonstrated an unusually bright, irregularly shaped structure in the center of the pocket, not visible on the first scan after her surgery.

The radiologist reading ultrasounds that day knew that something was clearly wrong, but she was not sure what the new abnormality was. "I've never seen an abscess look like this," she admitted. "I have no idea what that irregular bright area is within the fluid. I doubt it's a tumor, if the ovaries looked normal five months ago, but a case this unusual deserves a CT scan for some more info."

Had the post-operative abdominal x-ray film in the hospital been positioned properly, or been repeated as recommended, the diagnosis could have easily been made right after surgery, without the woman having to bear worsening discomfort for five additional months. Unfortunately, a series of missteps had occurred, and this unfortunate woman suffered the consequences. The CT scan done later that day unequivocally confirmed the nature of the abnormal ultrasound finding. A surgical sponge was retained within her pelvis.

Scrub nurses in operating rooms routinely perform a sponge and instrument count during surgical procedures, in order to account for all of the items set out for use during the operation. Of course, people occasionally make mistakes in counting, and in urgent cases, there may not be time to count at all. Knowing this, manufacturers of surgical sponges weave fine metal threads into the fabric, so that a retained sponge will show up by x-ray. Only a small fraction of surgeries are complicated by retained sponges or instruments; yet given the sheer number of operations performed every day, mistakes are bound to happen sooner or later. Surgeons taking care of these patients have to consider the possibility of human error, including their own.

Like many people, this woman experienced an undesired consequence from her treatment. She underwent surgery in order to feel better, but temporarily endured an unplanned and unsuspected side effect after mistakes were made by the medical staff who had tried to help her. These people were almost certainly honest and hardworking, but less than thorough on that particular day. She had put her body, trust, and faith into the hands of skilled professionals, but the very doctors, nurses, and x-ray staff she looked to for help had unintentionally let her down, at least for a while.

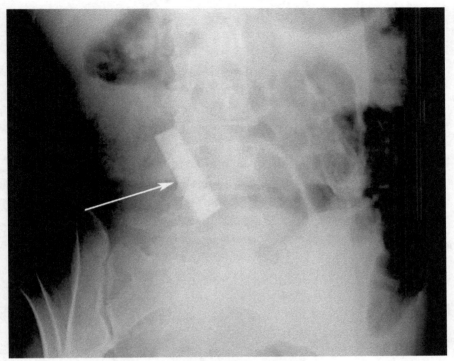

Retained surgical sponge
The labeled white rectangular structure in this patient's abdomen is a surgical sponge left behind during an operation. Metal fibers are woven into the sponge during manufacturing so that sponges retained during surgery can be detected by x-ray.

The gynecologist performing the hysterectomy had accidentally not retrieved one of the sponges. The operating room nurses did not perform an accurate count. The x-ray tech student took a substandard film and failed to repeat it. Both the radiologist and the x-ray supervisor failed to make the student repeat the film, and the OB residents who ordered the x-ray failed to request a repeat as well, despite the recommendation. Then the residents ordered a different test, an ultrasound, which is designed to detect problems other than the one the patient actually had. Finally, the suggested follow up scan was not ordered or scheduled in the recommended time frame, further delaying the diagnosis and prolonging the patient's discomfort. A proper surgical count—or a quick, inexpensive x-ray five months beforehand—could have prevented all of that.

When we finally got to look inside her adequately, we found the sponge. We also found a sequence of failures, in a system designed to prevent such outcomes. No single individual involved in the patient's care intended to do a bad job. All were working within a network of checks and confirmations, designed to prevent or catch errors. And yet, an error did occur, and went undetected for quite a while. The quality assurance chain had some weak links, and in her case, it broke.

A retained sponge may be debilitating, but it is fortunately usually more of a nuisance than a life-threatening emergency. The sponge was removed, and the woman got better. She also received an undisclosed out-of-court settlement from the hospital, and everyone involved learned something from the experience.

ABS OF STEEL

The young man reportedly could barely hold still while riding in the back of the ambulance, heading toward the city hospital late at night.

"Damn!" he shouted. "Aw, Jesus, I've been stabbed!" He reached for his abdomen, which was covered with a hastily placed bandage, now partially stained in blood.

The paramedics reassured him. "Hang in there, we'll be at the hospital in a couple of minutes."

Moments later the ambulance pulled into the entrance of the emergency room. A crowd of emergency physicians and surgeons, at various levels in their training, crowded around the stretcher to hear the report from the ambulance response team.

"Twenty-eight-year-old male, stab wound to the abdomen. The patient is alert and oriented, no loss of consciousness, Glasgow Coma Scale 15, complains of pain at the stab wound site, no other complaints. Blood pressure 135/80, pulse 96, pulse ox 99% on room air. No other signs of trauma. Bleeding at the wound appears relatively mild. Incident details unclear; the perpetrator fled the scene of the crime, as did the victim's friend who called 911. Police are still investigating, but the weapon was not found."

"What are you all going to do to me?" the thin, dark, young man said with fear in his eyes.

"We're going to look after you," the doctor in charge said. "You're here at the hospital."

"I know that!" he replied.

"Can you tell us what happened?" the doctor asked.

"Man, I don't even know, but some dude jumped me and stabbed me right here." He gestured toward his bloody abdominal bandage, which was being removed by a resident. "Ouch, be careful, that hurts!"

"We've got to see the stab site. What were you doing before the stabbing?" asked the doctor.

"I wasn't doing nothing," he said. "I don't even know who the hell it was. What you gonna do to me?"

"We'll let you know after we check you out," he said. "We're going to take care of you."

They examined him and saw no other injuries.

"Are you in some kind of gang?" one doctor asked.

"No man, I ain't in no gang," he denied, looking away.

"So what were you doing out at this time of night where somebody would try to stab you?" he asked.

"Man, I don't know, I was just in the wrong neighborhood. I wasn't doing nothing. Damn this hurts!"

The young fellow was not convincing in his story, but he was found to be sober, with no drugs in his system.

"What do you think—CT or DPL?" a trauma surgeon asked a resident.

"One puncture site, no other distracting injury, vital signs stable—I vote for a DPL," he said.

"Let's do it," commanded the doctor in charge.

"What's that? What are you gonna do to me now?" the patient shouted.

"Just try to relax and hold still for a few minutes," said the doctor. "We need to see if you've been hurt on the inside."

The doctors performed the procedure, known as a diagnostic peritoneal lavage, by cutting a small hole into his abdominal cavity, pouring in sterile saline, and suctioning back the fluid. If the aspirated fluid contains intestinal contents, that would indicate that the bowel has been perforated, and the patient would be taken to surgery. If the fluid shows a large amount of blood, then a significant injury such as an organ laceration would be suspected, and surgery might also be indicated.

In the past, blood would have almost definitely meant surgical exploration, but that approach has changed thanks to imaging. Not every injury that causes internal bleeding requires surgery.

Sometimes the bleeding stops spontaneously, and the patient can simply be observed in the hospital and released when stable. In addition, not every substantial internal injury results in blood or bowel contents entering the abdominal cavity. Because a deep peritoneal lavage may miss an important injury, or may detect signs of internal trauma that is genuine but does not require surgery, deep peritoneal lavage procedures are done less today than in years past, having been replaced primarily by CT scans to evaluate for internal injury.

On that particular night, this young man's deep peritoneal lavage fluid was clean. With no evidence for any internal injury, he had his wound stitched, was observed overnight, and released the next day.

He came back to the hospital clinic five weeks later, complaining of worsening abdominal pain ever since the stabbing.

"What seems to be the problem?" the clinic doctor asked him.

"My stomach still hurts," he told her, more subdued than during his emergency room visit weeks earlier. "It never stopped hurting, ever since I got stabbed. It's just not right."

"When does it hurt the most? Only at certain times?" she asked.

"Sometimes worse than others, but it hurts all the time, really. Sometimes it hurts to move, or to lift anything. It's painful, and it's making me weak." His former tough, street-wise demeanor had been partially replaced with meek uncertainty. On the night of his stabbing he was dethroned from youthful invincibility. Now he was reluctantly but admittedly needy.

"Where exactly does it hurt?" she asked.

"All over in here," he gestured, rubbing his hand over his mid-abdomen. She examined him. His scar had healed and did not look infected. Gently she placed her hands on his abdomen. It was flat, thin, and not distended. He was lean, and his abdominal musculature was naturally firm at his young age.

"All in there is where it hurts," he reiterated, mildly grimacing.

She ordered an ultrasound to look at his abdomen. It may not have been the best study to order, but she probably figured that it was not a bad place to start. Ultrasound is usually faster and cheaper than a CT scan. She had low expectations of finding anything anyway, given that five weeks had passed since the assault, and no internal injury was confirmed the night of the attack.

The ultrasound showed no internal fluid to suggest blood. His liver, spleen, and kidneys looked normal. However, one thing was out of the ordinary. The tissue at his stab scar was harder to see through than usual. The ultrasound waves did not penetrate through a region across his abdominal muscles, preventing us from being able to see anything deep to this spot. More unusual still was that the portion we could not see through had a perfectly straight margin on some of the pictures. Perfectly straight lines rarely occur within the human body.

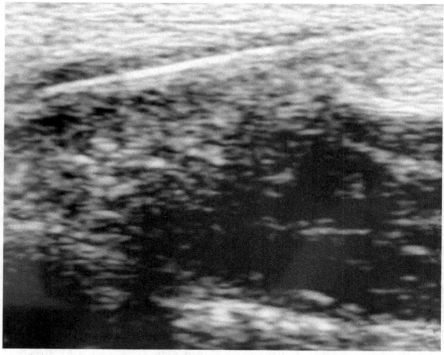

Abdominal ultrasound image showing an unexpected diagonal white line

Confused by the ultrasound images, we wondered what might cause a long, perfectly straight line to show up in the man's abdominal wall, blocking sound waves. The sharp line was reproducible, persistent with additional scanning, not some sort of unusual technical artifact. Perhaps scar tissue had formed along the puncture site. Alternatively, it was unlikely but possible that the doctors performing his incision a few weeks prior had accidentally left behind an instrument that might explain the unusual findings. Although this scenario was highly unlikely, we sent the young man down the hall for a single, inexpensive x-ray of his abdomen.

Minutes later the x-ray tech and another radiology resident in the program brought me the young man's abdominal x-ray film. Both of them were smiling.

"I think we have a diagnosis," the resident said, handing me the film.

I held it up to the view box lights. "Oh, my God!" I uttered in disbelief. "You've got to be kidding!"

"Can you believe it?" she beamed.

"No!" I said. "For five weeks this thing has been there!"

"I thought I'd seen it all at this hospital," the x-ray tech said, "but this is a new one on me."

The x-ray film showed something far more improbable than a retained medical instrument. A five-inch metal knife blade projected across his abdomen. It was not visible on the outside of his skin.

"The knife is still inside of him!"

Rather than being stabbed such that the knife tip went deep into his abdominal cavity, next to his organs and intestines, his assailant had placed the knife horizontally within the young man's abdominal muscles. Either the attacker came from the side, or the patient turned sideways at the moment of impact. Regardless, the entire knife blade had broken off from its handle, penetrated the tissue past its depth, and lodged in his abdomen.

We broke the news to him. He was understandably animated on hearing his diagnosis.

"You mean to tell me I still got the blade in there? The *knife* is still in me?! Oh, hell, I ain't believing this!"

Evidently he had not been required to pass through any metal detector since his stabbing, or the diagnosis could have been made sooner. He had walked around for five weeks with that knife blade embedded in his abdominal wall muscles. The surgeons removed it, and he recuperated uneventfully.

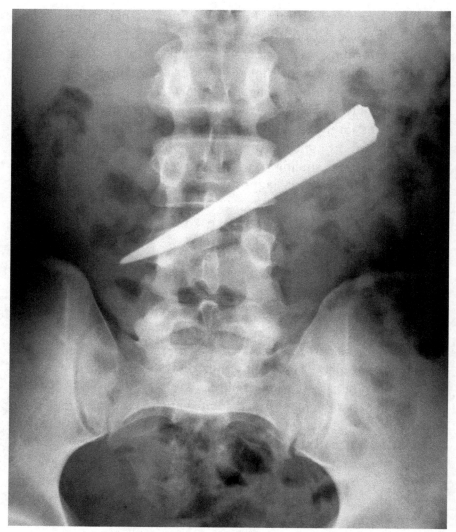

X-ray image of the knife blade within the patient's abdomen

This is where the story ended, or so I thought for nearly two decades. It was certainly interesting enough that someone could unknowingly have a large knife blade inside of him for so long, but the tale and x-ray held no obvious moral message, other than the observation that even a tough, healthy youth can succumb to injury or illness. He survived with no lasting damage, and there was an oddly amusing disbelief for anyone looking at the x-ray with that knife.

However, what I discovered years later was anything but funny. Before finalizing this book, it occurred to me on a whim to do a quick internet search, to see if I could learn whatever happened to this man after the incident.

I have no direct knowledge what his life was like for a number of years after his stabbing and the discovery of the embedded knife, but there must have been plenty of other trouble. The internet search revealed that, not long before this book was completed, the now middle-aged man was sentenced to life in prison, convicted of murdering his considerably younger girlfriend. While the couple lay in bed one evening in their apartment, he shot her, possibly under the influence of drugs, and then he fell asleep. Her mother was unable to reach the young woman the next day, so she came by the apartment and found her daughter dead, the perpetrator still passed out and lying on top of the victim.

Now with knowledge of this tragedy, I see the x-ray in a whole new light. When we see the outline of that cold steel, we are reminded of the devastating consequences of violence. The future might have been so different for a little girl unknown to the stabbing victim at that time—a child then, who would become his lover years later. His stab wound was not serious, and he lived; and because he did survive, she later did not.

Au Naturel

The MRI technologist called me on the phone. "Can you please come talk to my next patient? She's here for an MRI of her liver, but she doesn't want the contrast."

I stepped out of my dark reading room and walked down the hall into the technologist's control room. Looking through the glass window into the scanning room, I saw the patient, the one living entity in an otherwise stark room. The walls and floor were white and smooth, unadorned and clean. The patient, in contrast, wore rings on several fingers, visible as her arms were crossed, and her hands gripped her toned biceps. She leaned against the MRI table, which was sticking out from the cylindrical machine. Her long legs made the light blue hospital gown she was wearing look like a mini-dress. She was in her mid-forties but looked younger. Her brown hair cascaded over her shoulders. She was attractive, but her expression was slightly perturbed.

I read her doctor's order. She had recently had an ultrasound for pain in her upper abdomen, and that study revealed no gallstones. However, it did find an area in her liver that was probably a common benign tumor, which the MRI would clarify. She had no other current illnesses, and no history of cancer.

Given the strength of the MRI magnet, I removed the keys and coins from my pocket per standard protocol, took off my pager, and laid my wallet on the counter in the control room, so that my credit and ATM cards would not become demagnetized and rendered inactive. I then stepped into the magnet room and introduced myself. The woman was polite, but after our introduction, her more assertive side took control.

"So what's this chemical you want to put in me?" she quizzed. "My doctor didn't say anything about getting an injection."

"I'm sorry he did not mention that part of the study, and that this is a surprise to you, but he did order it that way. There is a reason for injecting contrast. It lights up the blood vessels, and shows blood flow to the lesion in your liver."

"My doctor didn't say anything about it. He just said there was an area in my liver that showed up on my ultrasound, and that I needed the MRI to see what it is."

"That's right. And the MRI pictures will tell us a lot more about the lesion if we can see the blood flow to it."

"What exactly is the stuff?" she asked. "I presume it's something artificial made in a lab."

"It contains gadolinium, a natural element from the earth that shows up under the magnet. It's been put it into a compound that can safely travel through the bloodstream. "

"Great," she replied sarcastically. "It's bad enough that I couldn't eat before coming, and that I have to go into that narrow tunnel. Now you all may be poisoning me."

I took a breath before speaking too defensively. "We're definitely not trying to poison you. In fact we're simply trying to do as good a study as we can, in order to make a diagnosis. If this lesion looks benign, you might be able to ignore it in the future, or at least follow it less frequently. Plus a good diagnostic study may avoid the need to consider a biopsy—something we do all the time if somebody needs it, but that could be riskier and more painful than an injection."

She looked at me warily, with just a hint of smile that was hard to read.

"I've had the injection myself once," I admitted. "Didn't even feel it. Most patients have no trouble with it. It really is quite safe."

My answer did not appease her. While remaining courteous, she proceeded to describe her philosophy on avoiding artificial substances.

"I'm not comfortable with it," she began. "I'm not into things that aren't natural. I take no medication, only herbal supplements, plus vitamins, and eat very well. I do get my checkups every year, but believe in prevention, and think you doctors sometimes could learn a little more about natural remedies and alternative treatments."

"Prevention is great, and I'm a believer in whatever works," I interrupted, in general agreement with her philosophy, though refraining from pointing out that the terms *herbal* and *natural* may also be used to describe hemlock and poison ivy.

She continued without missing a beat. "I exercise regularly, drink only a little wine, and haven't smoked in years. I don't like anything artificial—sweeteners, preservatives, or drugs. I haven't had so much as an aspirin in months."

The technologist looked at the clock on the wall, then at me, signaling concern about her patient schedule backing up. I wanted to get back to the issue of the injection.

"I'm just telling you why I'm hesitant. I believe in maintaining the natural state of my body, and am not interested in receiving anything artificial if I can help it," she concluded.

Although a little frustrated, I saw her point, and was becoming resigned to the situation. I remembered once giving a talk on all of the drugs that had led to emergency room visits or hospitalizations during my year of internship, and it was a surprisingly high number of medications. Side effects from any approved drug are usually fairly rare, but hardly nonexistent. Still believing that the MRI contrast injection is very safe, I thought she may have been overreacting, but I could relate to her position and to her fear of the unknown.

Based on her ultrasound and her history, the odds were that her liver lesion was benign anyway. We could get some useful information without an IV injection, and if the mass looked probably benign, we could always just follow it periodically to make sure it did not grow or change any further.

"I get it, and all of that is fine," I said. "I firmly support people being in charge of their lives and living healthfully. With regard to this test, all I can tell you is that we will get more information, and be able to make a more accurate diagnosis for you, if you were to get the IV injection. I certainly cannot make you take it if you don't want to, and would not try to do that. However, you need to know that the study will not be as thorough without the injection. It will definitely be better than nothing, just not complete."

"I appreciate that, but I'm going to pass on having that put into my body," she exclaimed. "I know you're just trying to do your job, but I don't want that chemical inside of me."

"That's fine. We can go ahead and do the part without the injection, and see how everything looks, then follow it down the road, particularly if it looks as if it's probably benign."

The technologist had the patient recline and positioned the sliding table within the machine. I watched on the monitor from within the control room as the first image of the woman's lower chest and upper abdomen came into view.

When I saw the first picture, I paused, smiled, and then shook my head while recalling our preceding discussion. The woman had breast implants.

Her liver mass appeared to be a hemangioma, the most common benign solid liver lesion, and it did not enlarge on subsequent studies over the following year or two.

In addition, her concern of minimizing foreign material in her body was eventually validated somewhat, despite the irony of her own implants. Within less than a decade since her study, the contrast that we formerly used indiscriminately—almost always with no complication—was discovered to cause a rare but serious soft tissue hardening phenomenon in a small percentage of patients with kidney failure, a condition known as nephrogenic systemic fibrosis. So nowadays MRI contrast is typically not given to patients with impaired kidneys below a certain level of function.

And, only a few years ago, it was discovered that patients who have received past injections of MRI contrast may end up getting deposits of the gadolinium in body tissues, including the tissue that lines the brain. The clinical significance is still being studied. There may be no adverse consequence whatsoever. Nevertheless, her story and these subsequent discoveries some years later remind us yet again that we often do not know all that we think we do....

HARD TO SWALLOW

The bearded, bespectacled physician from the emergency room patiently stood in the entrance to my reading room on a Friday evening. Holding a microphone, I finished dictating a case with one hand and waved him in with the other.

"I know you're busy," he said politely, "because we are. My question should be quick." I typed his patient's name into my computer, and we found her CT scan on my ever-growing list of studies to read.

"The scan was done a few minutes ago, and I just looked at it on our monitor before walking over here," he explained. "I didn't see anything. Yet she seems like a reliable person with a straightforward story. She's a previously healthy young woman with an upset stomach, and she thought she would feel better if she made herself throw up. So, she tried to induce vomiting with her toothbrush, but somehow let go. She says she swallowed it."

"Wow, that happened to a girl I knew in college," I said. "I'm surprised to hear that history twice in a lifetime—although there was more to that story, which I can tell you when we're done with this one."

"It's a new one for me," he admitted. "First we got x-rays of her chest and abdomen, but your colleague down the hall didn't see anything, and the x-rays do look normal. Yet the patient was so certain that she accidentally swallowed it that I felt compelled to get the CT. I still don't see anything, even though she swears it ought to be there."

I first clicked open the chest x-ray image on my computer screen, then the abdominal x-ray. He was right: if there was a toothbrush in there, it was completely invisible.

"These do look normal," I agreed. "But the CT ought to show *something*."

Nevertheless, when we began reviewing the cross-section CT images one by one, nothing visibly jumped out at us. Her stomach was nearly empty, containing a very small amount of normal fluid, plus what looked like a little debris with gas in it, presumably the residual of whatever she last ate. And yet, something did not seem quite right, although I could not exactly pinpoint just what it was. I had the strange feeling that something could be hiding right before our eyes. We would be doing her a disservice if we missed it.

"I don't see anything obvious," I said.

"No, neither did I, which is why I came over here to ask your opinion. She seemed certain. Is it possible she's mistaken somehow?"

"Let's look at these coronal and sagittal images," I said. In addition to the standard horizontal images, the technologist had been thorough and had used the computerized scan data to generate other pictures from different projections through this woman's abdomen. Having failed to find anything by looking from top to bottom, we then examined her organs from frontal and side views. Still there was no clear sign of a toothbrush—but something gnawed at me.

"Would it be obvious if it were there?" he asked.

"I would have thought so. Granted, I've never seen this before, on x-ray or CT, but usually a foreign body that size would stand out. We know that kidney stones we can't see on plain x-ray still look bright on CT, so I thought maybe a toothbrush might at least look slightly bright. Clearly we don't see anything like that."

"It must depend on what something's made of," he said.

"That's true. I'm sorry, I just don't see it."

"No, me neither," he said, bewildered, "but it's a confusing story. I'm not sure what to do next. If we can't confirm it's there, then I'm not sure there's any point in calling in the gastroenterologist on call."

He thanked me and went back to the emergency room. I remained perplexed by the disconnect between her story and her scan, but proceeded to review the rest of the images, in order to dictate a report and move on to the next case. Something still seemed off to me on some level. There was one more set of pictures that we had not yet looked at, and when I opened that series up, my first reaction was mild annoyance.

"What the heck are these?" I mumbled to myself, wondering why the technologist had generated a set of pictures that were not at all a conventional view, and why he had not recognized his mistake before permanently storing them in the computerized x-ray system. Reflexively I picked up the phone and dialed the tech at the CT scanner, hoping he might be able to delete them, while briefly scrolling through what I thought would be garbage images.

They turned out to be the most important pictures the technologist generated, earning him my further respect, helping us treat the young woman, while helping me and the emergency doctor save our reputations.

Literally as the phone was ringing and I half-heartedly skimmed pictures I thought had been made in error, I saw an even row of bristles in the upper part of the stomach, projecting from the end of a slightly curved handle pointed toward the lower stomach, near the outlet to the small intestine. It was unmistakably a toothbrush.

Its plastic handle contained air bubbles by design, for the manufacturer to use less plastic material in production. In the light of day it was a solid object, but the low density of the plastic embedded with air bubbles was completely imperceptible on the initial x-rays, and mimicked the appearance of swallowed food on the CT scan. Only then did everything become clear from these images obtained at an unusual angle, from the bottom right to the upper left, parallel to the natural position of the stomach.

What had bothered me about the standard-view images finally hit me: next to what had looked like food mixed with air was a normal uniform pocket of swallowed air in the stomach, separate and too distinct if her stomach had contained only normal food. Furthermore, the stomach was stretched long but thin, not contracted as when empty, nor rounded and evenly distended in all directions as when full. The toothbrush was lodged in her stomach, stretching its length, and there was no way it could safely pass further.

John, the CT tech on duty at the emergency room scanner, answered the phone. "I bet I know which case you're calling about," he said half-jokingly.

"You know it—the toothbrush," I admitted. "I was going to ask you what the heck that last series was, until I realized that you just saved the day."

"Yeah, I thought that oblique set showed it best," he said.

"It's the only one that showed it at all," I agreed. "Although in retrospect..."

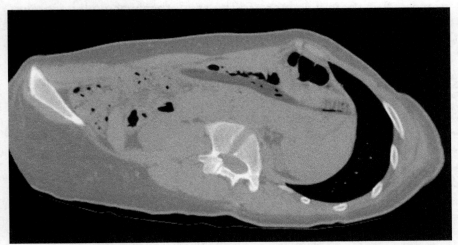

Swallowed toothbrush

"Yeah, I knew something didn't add up," he said humbly. "She seemed like a reliable person when she told me her story, so I figured it must be in there somewhere."

With that note, he brought the personhood of the patient back to mind. Upon mentioning the woman he had scanned and spoken with, she came to life a bit for me, and I felt empathy. No longer was she just represented by a series of cold, black-and-white pictures of her stomach. She was a real young woman who needed help—even though I never did meet her, hear her voice, or see her face.

"John, you get a gold star tonight. Thank you for using your head and saving my you-know-what. Now I've got to call that ER doc back and help him look good, too."

Immediately I called the emergency physician, told him the news, and asked him to come back to the reading room if he could. He arrived quickly, eager to see the elusive toothbrush.

"There it is," I pointed to the screen, as we reviewed John's unconventional oblique images through the plane of her stomach.

"Wow," he smiled. "That's amazing!"

It was. First, it was amazing that someone could actually swallow a whole toothbrush, but it was also amazing that we had so much trouble finding it, and that we almost missed it in the process. But there was more to the story that was now becoming complete before my eyes. I thought of a girl from school, and of internalized pain, and hidden behavior patterns. Like that toothbrush, the patient's secret was finally being revealed. When I looked at the screen, I no longer saw just a swallowed object; I envisioned a troubled person.

"She's bulimic," I said.

"Pardon me?" he asked in surprise.

"She's bulimic," I reiterated. "I told you that I knew someone else this happened to, back in college, only I learned about it some years later. Exact same story—she was using her toothbrush to throw up, but she got carried away and accidentally swallowed it. Think about it: if you wanted to make yourself sick, wouldn't you just put your finger down your throat?"

"Sure, I suppose," he said. "But she wasn't getting the relief she wanted."

"That's because she's deadened her gag reflex from doing this repeatedly. Now she's using an object to reach farther down her throat, trying to stimulate a reflex that is harder to trigger. Plus, look at the position of the toothbrush: she swallowed the handle end first. You would think that most people doing this the first time would place the bristle end first, like you're brushing your teeth. If she needs more than that to get an effect, she's done this a number of times."

"That's very interesting," he said, staring at the screen in thought.

"It may sound anecdotal, but this is not an isolated occurrence, and a story like that sticks with you," I said. "Hang on, I bet I can find an article to back this up." Turning toward a different computer, I did a quick literature search. Two articles quickly popped up, one in a radiology journal, the other reference in a pediatric journal, both supporting the assertion that a swallowed toothbrush is an indicator of bulimia.

"You better go ahead and line up a gastroenterologist to scope her," I said. "They should be able to retrieve it. That's what happened with my friend years ago. They got it out and spared her from needing surgery."

"I'm on it right now," he said. "Thank you."

"You can thank John on the CT scanner," I said. "I'd gladly go with you to talk with the patient about this, but I'm behind as it is, and don't want the rest of your colleagues mad at me if their other studies don't get read soon. Let me know what you find out."

The evening's work never subsided long enough for me to leave my desk, so I never got to meet the woman, who was taken for an upper endoscopy with sedation. The gastroenterologist was able to pass a scope into her stomach. Using a snaring device to grab the toothbrush, he pulled it back up the esophagus and out of the patient's mouth. She recovered from the extraction procedure fine, spared from open surgery.

Concerned about her, I tried calling her at home over the next several days, but she never answered her telephone. A week later I called the gastroenterologist for an update.

"I'm calling about a patient I'm sure you'll remember," I began. "The woman who swallowed her toothbrush."

"Oh yes," he immediately replied. "That was interesting. A little challenging to get around the bend in her throat, but we did it. Thank goodness for anesthesia."

"I didn't get to meet her, but I wonder if you had a chance to ask her about bulimia, which I referenced in her CT report."

"I did," he said. "She denied it. I wasn't convinced. She sort of looked away, and she kept saying 'no'. But, later on her boyfriend told me outside the room that she probably is. He said he's suspected for some time that she was doing that."

The boyfriend's suspicions, and the woman's denial, did not surprise me. Nor did it surprise me that I never got past her voice mail greeting when I called to see if she needed any recommendations for support. In her isolation, and probable embarrassment, she may avoid calls in general, particularly those she could identify as coming from the hospital where she had an unpleasant experience she would just as soon forget. However, I did not forget her. I can only believe that she has painful issues that need to be dealt with— and until she does, I fear that she will continue a behavior that may slowly but steadily damage her body and her mental health; and that really is hard to swallow.

Special thanks to John Fagan, RT-CT.
Image used from case report, Ruff C: "Swallowed Toothbrush—Bulimia," American College of Radiology, *Case in Point*, 23 Dec 2014.

THE MULE

O riginally from Mexico, the man in his early thirties was already under an unspecified degree of surveillance by the U.S. federal government, according to the surgeon anyway. Suspicions may have arisen from the young man's frequent travel between southern California and Washington, DC, perhaps because the man also had no identifiable work or family visits to explain his recurring transcontinental trips. Maybe it was because he could not demonstrate the income source for the airfare. Or, perhaps suspicions were raised from the discovery that a third party was buying his frequent airline tickets for him. For whatever reasons, he was to some degree already on the radar of the U.S. Drug Enforcement Agency (DEA). When he came to the hospital emergency room complaining of abdominal pain and swelling, it did not take long for federal agents to become involved in his case. That case got particularly interesting when the ER doctors ordered an abdominal x-ray to see if the man might have an intestinal obstruction. The x-ray image told a richer but disturbing story.

Indeed he did have a blockage of his bowel, but the reason was far from ordinary. Bowel obstructions are commonly caused by adhesions, bands of scar tissue that can form after surgery, or after an abdominal infection, restricting the bowel's normal motion and propulsion. Yet this man had had no prior surgery or known infection. What then was causing his obstruction, impairing his intestinal function to the point that he was no longer able to defecate, not even passing gas, with his abdomen becoming painfully and dangerously distended?

The x-ray revealed numerous non-metallic rectangular or cylindrically shaped structures, outlined by sharp margins, scattered throughout his small bowel. Again, perfectly straight lines rarely occur in the human body. Having so many of them appearing to be so well delineated throughout his abnormally dilated intestinal tract was not only unusual; it was highly suspicious.

The police sometimes accompany patients involved in motor vehicle crashes, assaults, and other such events, when people coming to the hospital may be under arrest with charges pending. But never had the surgeon or I seen authorities use such swift action in taking over the management of a patient likely heading to surgery after a diagnostic x-ray study. Nor had we ever dealt with federal DEA agents.

Again, the x-ray revealed multiple foreign bodies in the intestine. The structures were all the same size, each about two inches long. They were all filled with cocaine.

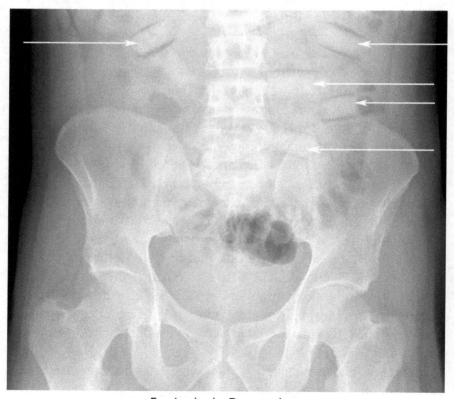

Foreign body: Drug packets
Swallowed packets of cocaine in the patient's intestines. (Dark areas on the image represent intestinal gas, some of which outlines the drug packets.)

Per the DEA surveillance, they suspected that on numerous occasions the man had swallowed multiple packets of drugs, boarded an airplane, arrived in another city, and gone to a place where he could wait until the packets passed, eliminated with his bowel movements. Then the packets would be washed, and the drugs would continue their journey, to dealers and ultimately to users. This time, however, he ran into problems. In addition to being under a greater degree of surveillance, with federal agents narrowing in on him as someone supplying drugs to the Washington, DC region, the man's intestinal tract could not handle the load he had ingested. He admitted to having swallowed sixty packets, but only thirty-nine passed while he was holed up, waiting to defecate the rest. He knew the exact number left to go, as did the people with whom he worked, because inventory that expensive has to be guarded and protected. The investment is costly, the street value too high, and the risks too great, not to capture all that went in before he boarded the airplane.

I did not meet the man, and with federal DEA agents involved, I did not risk overstepping my bounds by asking questions, despite understandable curiosity. Nevertheless, when looking at his abdominal x-ray and talking with the surgeon consulted, it was intriguing to think about the patient, the world in which he ran, and the circumstances and choices that led him there.

What must his life have been like to lead him to this point? How desperate must he have been, to risk his own bodily health and legal freedom in order to make money? Were his opportunities, his earning potential, so severely limited that it was worth taking the chance? Maybe he had developed a drug habit of his own, augmenting his own craving for money or drug resources, affecting his judgment, leading him to make worse decisions. Maybe he was in too deep by now to get out, feeling trapped in criminal life. Clearly the risk of getting caught must play into the equation—but caught he was.

Before coming to the emergency room, he apparently had waited until he could no longer stand the abdominal pain and distension. He may have even feared for the safety of any loved ones known to his supplier. Yet once it became clear that he was obstructed, and the drug packets would not pass, the fear of dying from the obstruction was greater than fears of legal repercussions. The instinct to live got him to the emergency room, even though he must have known that he would likely be arrested. The outcome and consequences would be disastrous for him as a free man, but he took his chances in order to stay alive.

Now he was going to earn nothing more, for years, and would find his circumstances more restricted than ever, as he joined the ranks of the convicted and incarcerated.

The surgeon took him to the operating room, made an incision, and found considerable scar tissue, causing a kinking of the small intestine near the connective tissue that lined his abdomen. Scarring is more common in people who have had prior abdominal surgery, which this man had not, and the surgeon theorized that perhaps repeatedly swallowing drug packets may have somehow damaged the man's intestines. The surgeon was able to dissect away the scar tissue from adjacent structures, and he then intentionally cut a hole into the small intestine, proceeding to milk the loops above and below the bowel incision, retrieving the drug packets that had not passed.

Twenty-one packets were removed, the exact number expected by the DEA agents standing in the operating room, ready to collect the drug packets immediately on removal. Each packet was wrapped tightly by a yellow plastic covering. None had ruptured inside the man. Had that occurred, some of the drugs would have been absorbed into his bloodstream, and the volume from even one packet could have been lethal.

The man went to prison, where he presumably remains. Maybe being convicted at least got him off drugs, if he is not acquiring them while incarcerated. And if he is no longer using and selling, maybe he can someday, somehow, make more of his life post-release, however far off in the future that may be.

After a few years in prison already, with more ahead, I wonder if he ever considers how many people, completely unknown to him, may have been adversely affected by his trade. How many users must have consumed the drugs that he helped make available by transporting them, defecating cocaine for eager buyers to purchase. For some users, the drugs were likely recreational, with no lasting consequences. But for addicts, and the people in their lives, the drugs' effects may have been more foul, infectious, toxic and wasteful than the excretory medium in which they were transported.

SECTION V: COMPLICATIONS

Errors in radiology come in different forms, and we have briefly explored a few in the preceding chapters. For the technologist, doing the correct study on the right patient, and doing it well, are paramount. For the radiologist, a fund of knowledge, visual perception and recognition, interpretation, judgment, and communication are all important components toward making diagnoses and effecting patient care. For the other physicians, assistants, and practitioners who order imaging studies or procedures on their patients, knowing which study to order and when, and on whom, are particularly relevant. There is no one best test for every diagnosis, or for every patient. The diseases or conditions under consideration are important elements in deciding which type of study may be most indicated. Sometimes the best additional test may be none at all.

Complications are another matter, and although they indicate an undesirable outcome, their occurrence may not always result from an identifiable error. Even when all of the steps are taken to perform a procedure correctly, to maximize outcome and minimize risk, adverse events may occasionally happen anyway, at times with devastating consequences. The highly acclaimed surgeon and writer Atul Gawande explored the subject of complications in his first collection of essays under that title, and other writers have addressed the subject from the perspectives of their own fields.

The examples in this section illustrate a few of the complications that may be encountered from interventional or diagnostic radiology tests, and they highlight some of the risks of undergoing some procedures in the first place. Signed papers of informed consent are more than a legal formality; they document our acknowledgement and understanding that, through no definite fault of any particular party, bad things sometimes happen to people, even though we seldom actually expect them to happen directly to us.

FLUSHED

"Check this out." The interventional radiology fellow pointed at the schedule of cases one morning during residency in 1996. "We're doing a carotid angiogram today on a thirty-five-year-old for hyperparathyroidism."

"Who the heck ordered that?" I asked in disbelief.

"Somebody who obviously needs to retire," he replied.

"Has her doctor never heard of a parathyroid scan?"

He shook his head. "The boss said they used to do these more routinely back in the day, and he approved it. He and the referring doc have known each other for years, and he wants to keep him happy. If she's got an adenoma, it should be hypervascular and show a blush."

The young woman's doctor suspected that she had a benign but hyperfunctioning tumor of a parathyroid gland, one of several very small glands on the back of the thyroid in the neck. An adenoma releases excess parathyroid hormone into the bloodstream, causing calcium to be removed from the bones, thus raising the blood calcium level, which can lead to complications including kidney stones and osteoporosis.

A nuclear medicine parathyroid scan would have been an easier, safer, and cheaper way to look for an adenoma, simply requiring an IV injection of a low dose radioactive substance taken up by parathyroid tissue. By comparison, the requested angiogram we were preparing to do was an older test, labor intensive, more expensive, not any more accurate, and slightly risky. It would require the puncture of the major groin artery with a needle, and the placement of a plastic catheter through that artery into her aorta, then up into her carotid arteries. An injection of iodine-based contrast would then light up the vessels, revealing increased blood flow to an adenoma, if she had one.

The case started off routinely, with the preparation, the needle and catheter placement, and the initial injections. At that point in residency, I had only a little experience doing angiograms, so I assisted both the attending professor and the interventional fellow doing his final year of specialty training. Being at the bottom of the physician totem pole in the x-ray procedure room known as the angio suite, my main job was to inject a small volume of sterile saline through the catheter on a frequent, regular basis to prevent a blood clot from forming on its tip. This duty meant that, at least during a procedure, the resident was known as "flush boy"—or, for a female resident, "flush girl."

The supervising radiologist who had approved the case, plus the fellow and I, a nurse and an x-ray tech, all stood around the patient lying on the table. All of us doing the case wore green surgical scrubs, with overlying lead aprons and sterile paper gowns. Each of us also wore a cap, a facemask, and goggles to protect our eyes from blood exposure. It got hot quickly.

The doctor teaching the procedure instructed: "OK, the catheter's in a good position. Let's see what we've got so far."

We filed out of the x-ray procedure room to the adjacent control room, briefly leaving the sedated patient on the table with the catheter in her groin. The x-ray tech had hooked an automatic contrast injector to the catheter. We stood behind the radiation-shielded window and watched as the iodine contrast was injected into her bloodstream, lighting up her arteries like a highway system. We had no idea that it would soon lead to a major detour.

"So far, so good," the fellow said. "Now we need to advance and select."

I kept up with the catheter flushes while they manipulated the catheter. A couple of more injections revealed that we were narrowing in on the artery supplying the parathyroid glands on her left side, but then the latest injection was completely unreadable, blurred from motion.

"Oh, for God sakes," the attending exclaimed. "She's moving all over the place. We've got to repeat that run." Walking back into the room, he advised the young patient. "It's really important that you hold still when we tell you."

"Are you still awake?" the nurse asked, checking to see if the sedative and narcotic she had given the patient earlier had suddenly become too powerful. "Hey?" She patted the woman's hand. Her eyes were rolled back. She moved slightly and moaned, but did not speak.

"Doctor, she doesn't look right. She wasn't like this at all a moment ago—you saw her, she was sedated but responsive."

"What the hell?" he said with alarm. "Speak to us. Are you OK?"

She did not reply.

"What are her vitals?" he asked, looking at the cardiac monitor while the nurse iterated the readings.

"Pulse ox is still 99%, normal sinus rhythm, blood pressure stable at 118/76."

"Did you give her any more sedation?" he asked.

"No, not since the last dose twenty minutes ago," she replied.

"Hey there, wake up, talk to us," he commanded. The patient moved about a little on the table but did not look at anyone directly or talk.

"Damn it, she better not have had a stroke. Get the hospital operator on the phone—I want whoever's on call for neurology to get down here immediately. Were you flushing the catheter?" he turned to me.

"Yes, the whole time," I said. The interventional fellow nodded in support. The look in his eyes was ominous.

Moments later a neurology resident entered the room. He was Asian, square-jawed and a bit heavy, early thirties, carrying an old-fashioned black doctor bag.

"What happened?" he asked.

"We're doing a carotid angiogram. She's had a sudden change in mental status and is very poorly responsive all of a sudden."

The neurologist took a few tools out of his pockets and black bag. He shined a penlight into her eyes, quickly checked her reflexes with a rubber hammer, poked the soles of her feet, and tried to get her to follow commands to check her strength and sensation.

"It's cortical," he said, surprised at his own findings and their implications. "She's had a stroke."

"Damn it," muttered the professor. "You're sure?"

"Yes, I'm afraid so," the neurologist said, checking a couple more reflexes.

"Thank you," he said. "All right, we don't have much time folks, let's get moving."

At first I had no idea what we were going to do next, and I was amazed to see that they were preparing for another injection, since our procedure had evidently caused her stroke. Again they gave her another iodine injection, but this time she held still just enough for the pictures to be interpretable.

"I think it's there," our professor said, pointing to the computer screen image. "Zoom in on this." Within the branching dark gray lines outlining her arteries, there was a little area in one branch artery to her brain that did not fill with blood.

"All right, let's select that branch," he commanded, again manipulating and advancing the catheter. Another moment and another small volume of contrast injected confirmed the diagnosis.

"That's it, for sure," he said, pointing to the latest run images on the screen. She had a blood clot in one of the artery branches to her brain. Despite the catheter flushing, a small clot had formed anyway, had broken loose and floated downstream to lodge into a cerebral artery.

"All right, let's get the urokinase ready folks," he ordered. The x-ray tech assisting with the procedure laid some plastic syringes of clear fluid onto the table. The doctor injected a small amount. "This better work."

He was starting over now, trying to reverse the outcome while he had a chance, attempting to wash away the damage done. The tension in the air was palpable.

After the first injection of the clot-dissolving drug, she was still clearly impaired. They repeated the contrast injection; the clot was smaller.

"Let's try to get out there a little farther and get as close to that thing as we can," he said, with perspiration collecting on his forehead. "Our best bet is to target the clot and get the urokinase right at it."

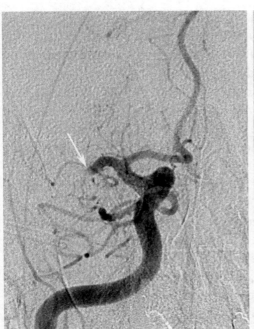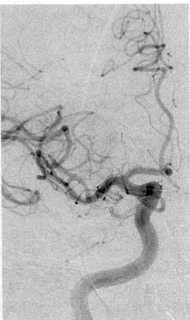

Embolic stroke
The dark material is iodine-based contrast opacifying arteries in a patient's brain. The image on the left shows a blood clot lodged in a cerebral artery blocking blood flow in a patient with stroke symptoms. The image on the right shows restoration of blood flow into the arterial branches downstream after blood clot removal.   —Images courtesy of Edward Greenberg, MD

With another injection of the blood-thinning medicine, the patient started to come around, and the clot was visibly smaller. After a third injection, it was no longer visible. Blood flowed through the widely opened artery and beyond. We paused, sweating, hoping, praying. Shortly afterward, she started answering questions.

"Can you hear me?" he asked.

"Yeah," she said drowsily.

"Do you hurt anywhere?" he asked.

"Huh? No, I'm all right. Maybe a little headache."

The nurse placed her fingers into the patient's hands. "Squeeze my fingers," she commanded. "Good. Equal grips."

"Wiggle your toes," the professor instructed. The woman did, equally on both sides. He continued a basic neurological examination; she passed each test.

"Unbelievable," I whispered to the fellow.

"Man, talk about pressure," he whispered back, too soft for the patient to hear. "You could have put a piece of charcoal up my ass a minute ago, and I would have spit out a diamond."

The patient remained conscious and showed no further or residual impairment.

"OK, we're done in here for today. Let's pull the catheter," the professor directed, then turned to the patient. "Do you remember any of what was going on during the past few minutes?"

"No," she denied, "I feel like I've been in a blur. I'm all right, though."

"That's what we're counting on," he replied, "but you've just bought yourself a night in the hospital, to make sure everything's all right. You had a close call there."

He turned to us. "Guys, she's going to need a head CT when we're done here, *now*, before she gets admitted. Let's make sure there's no sign of hemorrhage."

Her scan was normal. She had no bleeding in her brain, and no visible tissue damage. She was still a bit drowsy after the procedure, as she talked with her family in the hallway, but she was otherwise alert and oriented, with no residual deficit. We witnessed—we *caused*—an acute stroke in her brain, but fortunately immediate action dissolved the clot that would have left her permanently impaired. Learning how to dissolve a blood clot in an emergency was certainly educational, but the most valuable lesson for me was much more basic: we should have never done that procedure on her in the first place.

Later the young woman's mother and a couple of other family members stood by her stretcher. "If anything unusual can happen," her mother said, "this is the one it will happen to." The other family members teasingly nodded their heads, unaware just how close a call, and how serious a complication, she had really had.

They were also unaware of our strengthened resolve to serve the patient first while in our care, regardless of a referring doctor's request. I was already used to guiding other doctors who would ask which might be the best diagnostic studies to order for their patients, based on the patients' conditions, the information desired, radiation exposure, injection risk, and cost. Interventional procedural cases like this could have even greater potential for a bad outcome. Had she been left with a stroke, it would have mattered little to her that her other doctor had ordered the procedure, once the damage was done. We had agreed to do the test, despite the availability of safer and equally useful alternatives, and in the process of doing the requested procedure, had nearly left her permanently disabled. I would try my best to avoid going down that path in the future.

Editorial note: urokinase is a naturally occurring enzyme that helps dissolve blood clots. An alternative clot-dissolving drug more commonly used now is tissue plasminogen activator (tPA). In more recent years, blood clots, including those in arterial branches to the brain, may be treated with thrombectomy devices that directly remove harmful clots that impede blood flow, restoring normal blood circulation.

INSIDE OUT

The screaming from the nearby x-ray examination room was so loud that I was having trouble hearing the x-ray technologist talking to me.

"Our next patient will be ready in just a minute," she said over the cries of the woman in the next room. "She's been in the hospital for ages; we've done other studies on her. I know she's had complications after gastric bypass surgery, but I can't tell you much more than that. Her story sounds complicated. Her chart's right here if you want to look through it first."

"I do, but I'll try not to take too long, given the sounds of her."

"She's absolutely miserable," she emphasized, while the patient cried out again. "She's got awful pressure sores and is in extreme pain lying on the table, but we can't put much else underneath her in order to do the study. Anyway, the sooner we get her back to her room, the better."

"Honest to God," I agreed, during another wail from the next room.

I started to read the woman's voluminous chart, but found the process only mildly faster than trying to sift through *War and Peace* for the kernels of information I needed most. I paged the resident instead. The surgeons taking care of her had ordered a fistulogram, a type of x-ray injection that evaluates abnormalities in the abdomen that can form from surgery or inflammation.

"I'll be doing her fistulogram and was hoping you can give me a little more history."

"Absolutely," she said. "In fact I'll try to come down in a bit, I'd like to see what it looks like. She's got a complicated story, but the bottom line is that she had a gastric bypass with a roux-en-Y gastrojejunostomy about six months ago." The procedure is one of several methods of surgically reducing the size of the stomach. "She ended up having a postoperative leak. She had to go back for a repair, but it never healed well. Her abdominal wound was left open, and now she has three holes within the wound that are draining fluid. We think it's probably coming from her intestines and want to see where the connections are if possible."

"We'll give it a try," I said, as the patient in the next room cried out again in pain. "We don't have a nurse available for pain control. Any chance the woman's nurse could come down with a dose of something for her?"

"She got a shot of Dilaudid right before she got sent down," the young doctor said. "Pain control has been another one of her issues. I'm afraid her nurse is too busy with other patients to leave the floor."

A moment later I introduced myself to the patient, who was lying on the hard, cold x-ray table, cushioned with a foam pad and some folded sheets. Despite being a very large woman, she did not look quite so overly nourished as she presumably once was. She had a loose-skinned, flabby, ironically withered quality that had come from losing weight the hard way, by slow starvation combined with tissue breakdown from illness.

"I don't mean to be hollering like this," she cried, "but it's just so painful lying on my butt like this with these ulcers!"

"Please, you don't have to apologize," I said.

"I've been bedridden for so long. I'll try to cooperate as best as I can, I just don't know how much more of this I can take."

Her apology was sadly touching. She was not a malingerer seeking drugs, nor was she asking for undue sympathy. She was trying to alleviate our difficulties in treating her, despite the fact that she was the one who needed consoling.

"We're sorry you're in so much pain. We'll try to do your study quickly so you can get back to your room and rest afterward."

"Do what you have to do to get a good test," she cried, "because I don't want to have to go through this again."

"Absolutely. Just a few questions before we get started. I just spoke with one of your residents, who said your first surgery for the bypass was about six months ago?"

"Yes—and I've spent five of the past six months in the hospital, including a full month in the ICU. You name it, and it has gone wrong with me. I can't begin to tell you how horrible this whole ordeal has been, and still is."

"I need to see your wound before we get started." She nodded and raised the cotton gown that covered her protruding belly. On her abdomen was a pile of gauze held in place by white tape. I snapped on gloves and gently peeled back the tape, removed the outer dry gauze, then the deeper damp gauze, exposing an open area with no overlying skin, roughly eight inches wide by a foot long. There was no actual skin over her unhealed abdominal wound— only wet, beefy red granulation tissue that glistened under the fluorescent lights. The surface of the tissue was slightly bumpy, not perfectly smooth, having several small mounds of soft tissue with tiny openings leading deeper into her abdominal cavity.

"These tiny holes in your wound are draining a bit of fluid," I explained, but she already knew. "Most likely there's a separate track coursing from your intestines to each of these holes, called a fistula. I need to pass a thin tube into each one and gently inject some contrast under the x-ray, in order to see what these fistulas connect to. It shouldn't hurt much—in fact you may not feel it at all. Do you have any questions?"

"No," she winced again, "just get it over with."

One by one, I took a thin, flexible catheter, dipped the tip in lubricating gel, and introduced it into the three small holes within her open wound. The tube placements were not painful, despite the reddened, angry appearance of the tissue. Each time I passed the thin tube until it would go no farther, then injected contrast fluid while watching under x-ray. The tube injections revealed three separate tracks that led from the surface, deep down into her abdomen, where the fistulas eventually connected to three separate corresponding loops of small intestine.

The surgery and its complications had caused gastric acid and caustic bile to break down the integrity of the reconstructed bowel. The erosive fluids and inflammation had formed these fistulas that drained some of her intestinal fluid all the way to the exterior. The three distinct channels were far from being straight lines, but rather tortuous and irregular, as they crisscrossed her surgically altered abdomen toward the surface. Now a portion of what she ate and drank, as well as some of the digestive juices her body naturally produced, were pouring forth to irritate previously healthy tissue and leak out into the open.

"We've found what we need to see," I said to her, briefly explaining the study results.

"Please tell me I don't have to have another operation," she begged.

"I don't know if you do or not. Your surgeons will have a better idea. I'll be sure to go over these pictures with them later today."

"Thank you," she said, wiping a tear from her eye. "Again, I'm sorry to have been so much trouble." With more pain and a few more tears, the woman was moved onto a stretcher, and a transporter wheeled her back upstairs to the hospital room that she knew all too well.

The surgeon and the resident did come down shortly after the study to review the images. We looked at the sequence of computerized x-rays that showed the woman's surgical complications.

"This case is a nightmare," the surgeon exclaimed. "She's had poor wound healing, and it's just one thing after another. Every time one problem improves, something else goes wrong. Despite her size, she's actually quite malnourished now due to our inability to feed her, and the fact that she's slowly weeping fluid."

The resident agreed. "She's got low albumin, low total protein, anemia, you name it."

"Which means if we were to do anything new at this point, she may not heal well from that either," the surgeon sighed, staring at the films.

"So what do you think you'll do?" I asked. "Assuming you have to get these tracks closed if her wound is ever going to heal right."

"It would certainly help. Honestly, I don't know what the heck we're going to do." He looked to be out of options, and his frustration was palpable. His reputation in the local medical community was exemplary. He was experienced, dedicated, and kind, yet completely mystified at how to put her back together properly.

Even gastric bypass patients with better surgical outcomes than hers can still have a myriad of problems with nutrient absorption, vitamin deficiencies, chronic diarrhea, scar tissue formation, bowel obstructions, ulcers, and pain, whether in the initial recovery period or later down the line. Anyone in the business of weight loss surgery, formerly called bariatric surgery, knows of the complications that can result. The problem is that without doing something to alleviate their morbid obesity, these patients can be living time bombs with regard to their health.

For some folks who have been unsuccessful in losing weight by conventional methods, bariatric surgeries have become a more common remedy of last resort, often with impressive results. We know that maintaining a healthy weight is paramount in helping prevent or control a number of diseases, including diabetes, heart attack, and arthritis. We also know that, despite increased knowledge regarding nutrition and weight optimization, more people in countries of plenty are losing the battle of the bulge than ever before. The reasons are several-fold, and the challenge is admittedly harder for some than others. There are likely some hereditary factors, but before people passively accept their obesity as unavoidable due to genetics, they might first ask themselves if any of their own grandparents were obese to the same degree. Most were not.

Nevertheless, a progressively increasing number of people are undergoing gastric bypass operations. For most of us, our natural tendency when consenting to procedures with low risk is to trust that we will be in the majority who do well, suffering no significant complication. Much of the time, the decision to proceed is clear, when there is little alternative. The man who needs his appendix removed for appendicitis, or the woman who can no longer walk on an arthritic knee and is ready for a replacement, will understandably consent to surgery, even when aware of risks.

Some procedures, however, are more optional, cosmetic surgery being the most obvious. Although surgery is usually successful, and often life changing for patients, such procedures are certainly not without their share of uncommon but tragic complications. Would people considering gastric bypass still undergo surgery if they believed in the genuine possibility that they, personally, might actually suffer an outcome as horrendous as this woman's? And are the surgeons performing these procedures doing the ethical thing by operating on these people? The surgeons would undoubtedly declare that they are, backed by studies and statistics to make the claim. Most of their formerly morbidly obese patients live longer and healthier lives after having intestinal rearrangement, enjoying greater and longer lasting weight loss results than they ever had from their failed diet and exercise regimens. On the other hand, a small minority of patients suffer from bad outcomes of what might still be considered an optional operation.

I did not ask this woman her specific reasons for undergoing gastric bypass surgery. Most likely, her reasons were the same as everyone else's. She had desired an improved physical appearance, health, energy, and mobility. As a single woman, perhaps she also wanted to improve her opportunities for more physical companionship, or eventual partnering. As a result of her surgery, all of those desired goals became even more unattainable by the complications that left her sicker, weaker, immobilized, and more physically unappealing. She chose to have her gastrointestinal tract surgically rerouted, although her actual problem had lain not in the gastrointestinal tract itself. Now her main problem clearly was in her post-operative gastrointestinal system, only the surgeons had no clear way to fix the problem. Her "easy" way to attain health and beauty turned out to be anything but that. Lying in pain in the hospital for months, with a large open abdominal wound in front and decubitus ulcers in back, she would have given anything in order to get back the body she had decided to alter.

As soon as work was through that day, I called a dear friend of mine, a woman who has struggled with her weight all of her life.

"I can't divulge anything confidential regarding patients," I explained, "but please don't ever have gastric bypass. You would not believe the poor woman I met today, and the ordeal she is still going through, months after her surgery."

"Oh, no, I don't ever plan on doing that," my friend assured me.

But a few years later, my friend was heavier, more concerned for her health and future, and more desperate than ever. She decided to have the surgery.

I wanted to be supportive. I also wanted to understand why she changed her mind and was now willing to undergo the operation. Asking her directly, I listened.

"You have to understand addiction," she began, "and the reasons addictions get triggered. For me, the underlying problem was anxiety. As a small child, I learned to manage it with food. Unfortunately, there is no way a small child can anticipate that overeating leads to weight gain and other issues. Once this understanding took place, it was too late. The pattern was established and the cycle was in full swing. Once cravings begin, they can't always be controlled. That's why addiction is considered an illness. When complications like weight gain, the disapproval of others, and bullying occur, depression and self-loathing are added to the already complicated picture."

She continued. "Anxiety and depression have a familial component. These are complex issues that go way beyond living a healthy lifestyle. And in one way, food addiction is harder to kick than others. People can live just fine without drugs or alcohol in their life. I can't quit my addiction; I still have to eat to stay alive, but I have to manage it."

My friend had her surgery, and she never had a complication. The same thing happened with several other friends and acquaintances who have since had gastric bypass surgeries. All lost considerable weight, and most kept a lot of that weight off. Those who did not regain their weight are still heavy, but considerably less obese than before their surgeries.

However, even for those who recover well from the surgery, not everyone finds the long-term success they were seeking. One friend of mine who had gastric bypass unfortunately did eventually regain most of the weight she had lost after her surgery. Slow but steady ingestion of fattening food, sometimes even liquefying it to help get it down, allows people who crave calories to ingest them still, despite having a surgically reduced stomach and shortened small intestine. Despite imposed anatomical restrictions, the most important keys to weight loss success and maintenance may still ultimately be self-motivation and behavior modification.

More recently, I revisited these themes with my close friend who ended up having the surgery. She offered up further insight as I asked more questions.

"When I met that unfortunate patient doing that x-ray test, I described some of the complications she had. You understood how horrible it sounded for her. How did you go from never considering surgery, to deciding to proceed with it?" I asked in earnest.

"Because I was desperate," she admitted. "I was mentally, physically, and spiritually exhausted from a lifetime of fighting addiction, depression, anxiety, and self-loathing. I felt helpless and hopeless, with no other choices. I came to the realization that something had to change, or I was going to die. It was a very difficult decision for me to decide that risking death for a better life was a chance I wanted and needed to take. I did so, not just for myself, but also for family, because my illness affected them as well."

She explained that potential weight loss surgery patients undergo a psychological evaluation, to make sure they understand what they are getting into and what is necessary to succeed post-surgery. Required educational sessions cover possible complications. Nevertheless, her last comments on this topic were particularly poignant: "Most people probably don't think much about complications, but that may be true when contemplating any type of surgery, not just gastric bypass. Most people just hope and pray for the best. Complications only become real when they happen."

Back to the hospitalized patient in this story. More than a year passed since my initial encounter with that unfortunate woman. In that time I performed a lot more x-ray studies on people before or after surgery, and in the process met many more patients who underwent similar gastric bypass operations with good results, often losing over 100 pounds within the first year.

During the year since I met her, the woman in this story continued to be in and out of the hospital, still dealing with complications, still miserable on so many levels. She endured further complications from the fistulas that continued to drain fluid from her intestines to her abdominal surgical wound, preventing it from healing. Finally a colleague of the first surgeon was consulted, and was willing to take a chance on repairing the leaks with an additional operation. By that point the woman was miserable and desperate enough to go along with yet another surgery.

It worked. After an extended recovery, she eventually did get better, left the hospital, and did her best to reclaim her life. Her wound scars may look hellish, but not nearly so hellish as the ordeal she went through. She finally did make it out, alive, which had been no guarantee when we met.

For readers considering such a procedure, please remember that even a very small chance of a very bad outcome means just that: some unlucky individual may have a truly bad outcome. Most people in the hands of a good, experienced surgeon do well, and for many but not all, the results are long lasting. Yet for the admittedly small percentage of people who do not do well, the consequences may be devastating. When there is little choice, the decision to accept risk and proceed is easy. But when there is another option, I feel compelled to caution those who may consider undergoing elective surgery. Call it a gut instinct. May those who opt for surgery have the results they wish, with a speedy recovery, but please do your homework before making that decision.

"What a nightmare her case was," her surgeon admitted when discussing it again several years later. "Other than one patient who died, she was by far the worst complication we ever had."

Suggested resource: American Society for Metabolic and Bariatric Surgery, www.asmbs.org

Do No Harm

"**M**y brother has a little trouble with his short term memory," the woman explained. "But he understands why he's here. He lives with me and my husband."

Her brother looked older than his sister, but was actually younger, about sixty. She was well nourished; he was thinner, more haggard, with the lined face of a long-term cigarette smoker who liked more than an occasional cocktail.

"She's good to me," he said. "She takes good care of me."

"He's pretty easy," she said.

"You've had quite a year," I said, shifting the conversation to his medical history and the biopsy I was preparing to perform on him. "Your doctor told me that you had surgery for throat cancer about a year ago."

"You bet," he said, tracing his finger along a scar that coursed under his jaw and down his neck. "And radiation, too."

"My husband and I never could get him to stop smoking. But he was doing OK until his recent test results."

"I reviewed those this morning before you got to the hospital," I said, turning to face the man directly. "What did your doctor tell you?"

"He set me up to come in here and see you. He said you were going to put a needle in my lung."

"That's right," I agreed. "The CT scan showed that you have a new nodule in your lung that wasn't there a year ago. The PET scan you had last week tells us that the nodule is active."

"That's what the doctor said," his sister confirmed, "and that it could be a new cancer."

"It could. It could be a new lung cancer, or it might be a

metastasis from the throat cancer. The purpose of the biopsy is to tell the difference, because that would determine how this new tumor gets treated."

We went through the steps of a lung biopsy for the purpose of informed consent. He would lie face down on the CT table, and we would scan his chest. The pictures would guide me in placing a needle into the nodule toward the back of his lung, after giving him a pain killer and sedative. A pathologist would analyze the tissue.

We discussed the procedure risks. There was a chance he could bleed, and there was a very low chance of infection. He had about a fifty-fifty chance of getting an air leak inside the chest cavity from the lung puncture site, called a pneumothorax.

"Is that dangerous?" his sister asked.

"It can be, but usually not. Usually it's small, and you don't have to do anything about it. We watch you and get another x-ray in a couple of hours. If the air leak stays small on the x-rays, and you're doing all right, we let you go home after a couple of hours. Less than one person out of twenty has an air leak big enough to need a tube placed in the chest, to re-inflate the lung and let it heal. If that happens, you'll be spending the night in the hospital."

"I can handle those odds," he nodded. His sister smiled.

"Good. We try to control any pain with the medicine you'll get from the nurse."

"I'm all for that," he smiled.

"Most people are," I smiled back. "Very rarely could anything else occur, and if so, we'd treat it as best as we could. Any questions?"

"No, I think you've explained it," he said, reaching for the pen to sign the consent paper.

"Thank you," she said, looking more relieved.

"You're welcome," I said. "We'll do our best to look after him."

Little did any of us know what lay in store for him later that morning. His case would be anything but routine, and I would not have specifically explained all there was to know. He might not handle the odds after all, and those nice people would end up far from relieved. Very rare complications are sometimes so uncommon that even the doctor performing the procedure is barely aware of their existence, until they occur.

The biopsy began routinely. The nurse gave him a small sedative and pain medicine in his IV. The man held his breath when I asked him to and breathed quietly when I told him it was safe to do so. I placed the needle the first time and was only a few millimeters to the side of the small lung mass being targeted.

"Close," the CT tech said.

"Yeah, but not quite close enough," I countered, going back to reposition the needle slightly.

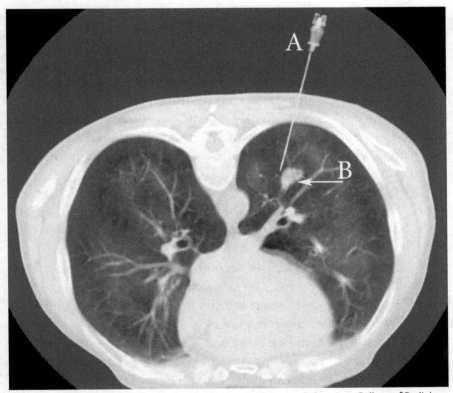

© American College of Radiology

Lung nodule biopsy, first pass
The biopsy needle (A) tip placed immediately next to the lung nodule (B).

The man held still. I pulled the needle back slightly, changed the angle, and re-advanced. His vital signs on the monitor were normal. The nurse and I stepped out of the room again and watched through the window, while the CT tech fired up her scanner and took another set of pictures.

"Bullseye," she said. The needle tip was right in the middle of the nodule. The lung had not collapsed at all. Vaguely and briefly, something on the monitor caught my attention, but only for a fleeting moment. The needle was right where it needed to be, and that pleased me, but the satisfaction quickly faded as we walked back in the room.

"Ow, oh," he groaned, "it hurts in my chest!"

"Toward your back, where the needle is?" I asked.

"No, in the front," he moaned.

"His rhythm is different," the nurse cautioned. I looked up at the monitor.

"His pulse is now 132. It looks like he might be going into V-tach," she said in a raised voice, meaning ventricular tachycardia, a rapid heart rate with a dangerous rhythm.

"Hang on!" I said, quickly taking one biopsy sample, then pulling the needle out of the man's back. "The needle's out, sir, we're done. Let's get you on your back." He was moving poorly. We rolled him over.

"Hand me a stethoscope. He didn't have a pneumo a second ago!" I listened to him breathe. Air entered both lungs equally. His heart beat too fast, his rhythm too wildly.

"He's in V-tach," the nurse reiterated.

"Call a code," I said. The tech grabbed the red telephone on the wall.

"His pressure and O2 sat are still normal," the nurse said.

"Give him more oxygen anyway," I said.

"I just did, he's on five liters and is at 99%," she explained.

"Sir, how are you feeling now?" I yelled. He barely responded.

"Sir, talk to us—does your chest still hurt? Talk to us! Damn it, what the heck is going on? Is he having an MI?!" I said, meaning a myocardial infarction, otherwise known as a heart attack.

Residents in white coats and surgical scrubs poured into the room. "I'm running the code team," one doctor announced. "What's going on?"

"I was doing a lung biopsy. He complained of sudden onset of anterior chest pain, not at the biopsy site. He got tachycardic, with probable V-tach. There was no pneumothorax a minute ago on the

CT, plus he's moving air on both sides, and his pulse ox and blood pressure have stayed normal. He's got no cardiac history, but he's a heavy smoker and could be having an MI."

"What was the biopsy for?" he asked.

"A new lung nodule. He had laryngeal cancer a year ago, or it may be lung cancer."

Several doctors were crowded around the man, assessing him in the resuscitation, preparing to give drugs and standing by with defibrillation paddles, ready to shock him if needed. The man's skin had turned from lightly tanned to ashen. He flinched only slightly when a resident dug her knuckles into his breastbone to check his level of consciousness.

"Let me check his scan once more while you guys are here," I said, quickly returning to the computer monitor outside the room. Another radiologist who had heard the resuscitation code announcement had just arrived, and was scrolling through the images on the screen while watching us from across the glass.

"I heard the code called," he said. "This is your lung biopsy? What happened?"

"Hell if I know," I said, briefly rehashing the events while we looked together at the images. "He doesn't have a pneumo at all. His coronaries are full of calcium. He could be having an MI, but why now?"

"Wait a second," he pointed, "what's this?"

There it was on the screen. It took a moment to register in our minds, and suddenly I realized that I had seen something subtly but dangerously different on his last images moments ago, when I was focused on the position of the needle tip. We were now staring at a life threatening complication that could kill him any minute, a complication that I had unknowingly and inadvertently caused, trying to help the man. It was so rare that, until that moment, neither of us had ever seen it, and barely remembered that it could even happen from doing a lung biopsy. I had not specifically warned the man or his sister that there was even a tiny chance that he could die from the procedure.

"Oh my God!" I exclaimed. "He's got air in his aorta—and his heart?!"

"Yeah, look," he pointed, detached from the emotion and commotion of the procedure room. "He's got air in his pulmonary veins here."

"Unbelievable. Absolutely *unbelievable*. He's got an air embolism."

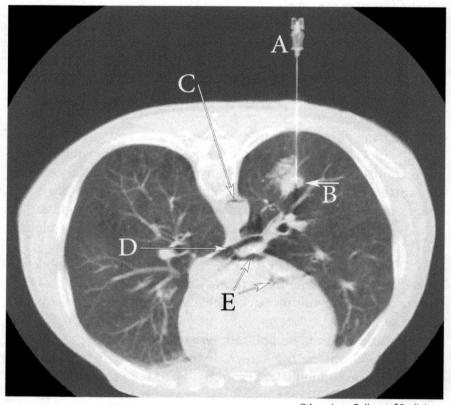

Air embolism

The tip of the biopsy needle (A) is placed into the lung nodule (B). Air is in the descending thoracic aorta (C), in a left pulmonary vein (D), and in the left atrium and ventricle (E).

"I think he had to," he said. "Somehow air got from the lung into a vein branch where you did your biopsy; then the air passed to his heart, and out his aorta." He scrolled back to the images after the needle was first placed, when the tip was close to the small mass but not quite in it. "Look, there was no air here before, but there is after you repositioned the needle tip."

There it was. Like a scuba diver who stays underwater too long and surfaces too rapidly, air had entered the man's bloodstream. The air bubbles could lodge in his arteries and block the flow of blood to critical organs, including his brain and his heart. The air could kill him right before our eyes by causing a stroke or a heart attack.

"I've never seen this. I was focused on the needle tip. I barely even had to reposition it. He was fine after the first pass. I only crossed the pleura one time. My God, have you ever seen this before?"

"No," he said. "But what else could it be?"

"Hold on," I said, hurrying back into the room where the team of doctors was still assessing the man. "He's got an air embolism!

He's got air in his left atrium and ventricle, and his aorta—put him in Trendelenberg position! Lower his head! Damn it, he'd better not be having a stroke and an MI both!" Residents quickly tilted the patient, moving his head lower than his feet, so that if the air left his heart it would be slightly more likely to travel away from his brain.

"His heart rhythm already reverted to normal," the doctor in charge of the code said. "We didn't have to defibrillate. He may be stabilizing." We then rolled the man onto his left side, to move his major coronary arteries lower than the dangerous bubbles in his heart chambers, still keeping his head down and his feet up. It may not have been much more sophisticated than a hope and a prayer, but those and the position changes were all we could offer at that moment.

"Let's get him to the ER," the chief commanded. The horde of young doctors wheeled the stretcher to the emergency department. I prayed that he would not be later wheeled to the morgue.

"His sister is still out in the hallway and is understandably confused and upset," the CT tech said. "Are you going to talk to her?"

I hesitated just slightly out of dread, but exited the door leading to the hallway. She sat alone in a small, exposed waiting area, wiping her eye with a tissue. She saw me coming to her.

"Doctor, what happened? What's wrong?" she implored as I

sat next to her.

"We did the procedure, and I got a piece of tissue, but there's been a complication, something I've never seen before. Some air got into his bloodstream from the biopsy, and it affected his heart."

"Is he going to be OK? I'm so scared!" She grabbed my hand.

"We don't know yet." I squeezed her hand back in return. "His heart rhythm changed temporarily, and he quit talking. I had to call a resuscitation code. They didn't have to do CPR or shock him, but he may have had a heart attack, maybe even a stroke."

"Oh, please God, no," she teared, her hands trembling.

"I'm so sorry," I continued. "His heart was doing better just a minute ago, and they took him to the emergency room. I'd like to go there now myself, to see how he's doing and make sure they have all the information we can tell them."

"Please, do whatever you can," she said, dabbing her eyes again.

The nurse reappeared. "You go on. I'll walk her over in a bit."

The man's heart rhythm remained normal, and his pulse had also slowed down to normal. Within a few minutes of arriving in the emergency room, he woke up. His mental status reverted to his usual baseline. He resumed talking normally. His memory was no worse than what it had been before we started, only he had no recollection of what happened after his chest had started hurting. He showed no sign of stroke, and his chest pain was gone.

When I later entered his room, the man was lying on his stretcher, still with his head lowered. He was casually talking with a nurse and a medical student.

"I can't tell you how happy I am to see you awake and talking," I said, grabbing his hand. "Don't sit up. Keep your head down. How are you feeling now?"

"OK, really. I feel fine," he said.

"Squeeze my fingers," I said, placing my fingers in each of his palms. He gripped them strongly and equally. He was able to move both arms and legs fine. He showed no sign of a stroke. The color and pulses were good in both hands and feet.

"We were really worried. You blacked out on us for a little bit there and gave us all quite a scare."

"I know," he said, "but I really don't remember much about it. Then I woke up here and all of these doctors were crowded around me. It kind of scared me."

"You're not the only one," I said, then tried to explain why it was important that he lie still. "You're definitely not going home today. We've got to watch you closely; you still may have had a heart attack."

"You think so?" he asked.

"Maybe. We have to wait and see. You look better now, for sure, but we need to keep a close eye on you."

Some of the residents and medical students who had been at his resuscitation code were talking at the nurses' station right outside the door. They had been looking up air embolism and its treatment. The young doctors had already contacted a local university with a hyperbaric chamber, a sealed room where the air pressure can be increased above normal, causing gas bubbles in the circulation to dissolve back into the blood. However, we ended up not needing to send the man over there. His heart rate and rhythm stayed normal, and he showed no sign of permanent damage. We did a CT scan of most of his body after a couple of hours, and the air in his bloodstream had been reabsorbed and had gone away. He showed no sign of stroke or other organ damage. He did get admitted to the hospital for a couple of days, but continued to do well and showed no evidence of an actual heart attack.

He got discharged and went home. A few days later I called to check on him and spoke to his sister on the telephone. By that point the biopsy result had come back, diagnosing a new lung cancer, caught early. He could be treated; the biopsy had been justified.

"It's not your fault," she said, ironically trying to comfort me. "I told my husband, I played bridge last night, and I got dealt a bad hand. That's just how it goes sometimes."

"I sure do appreciate your being so understanding," I thanked her. "I'm still just so glad that he came through."

"We all are," she said. "Thank you."

A surgeon removed the small lung cancer a few weeks later, and the man recovered uneventfully.

At the time of the biopsy, air must have entered one of his

coronary arteries, causing his arrhythmia and chest pain, but the bubble did not block the blood flow completely and permanently damage his heart muscle. His coronary event was fortunately temporary, but the lessons it had for the rest of us remain quite permanent.

(And even though I do not expect or hope to see this happen twice in my career, the consent form for lung biopsies has been modified to specify the possibility of this complication.)

Note: an earlier version of this story appeared in *Radiology Today* magazine, September 2008. Image used from case report, Ruff C, Urban B: "Air Embolism," American College of Radiology *Case in Point*, 1 July 2010.

SECTION VI: REFLECTIONS

My grandmother put it succinctly: "You can't beat Father Time." Try as we might to stay healthy and safe, we still know that ultimately something will get us. We will get sick, or hurt, and we will not be around forever. It may be quick, or it may be drawn out and gradual. We may have plenty of notice, or little warning at all. Yet although we know this intuitively, it is surprisingly easy to forget somehow, or to avoid thinking about until we have no choice. Maybe that's just as well on one level, allowing us to live more freely and unburdened while we can.

Although few diseases or accidents feel expected, they do often occur under somewhat predictable circumstances, depending on a person's age, heredity, living conditions, daily habits, and risk taking. Sometimes things happen unexpectedly, as statistical outliers or events of seemingly random bad luck. We search for meaning and explanation, but they are not always easily found. Despite having studied health and the human condition for over thirty years now, I regrettably have few answers to the questions that challenge us the most. No one comes out unscathed, but why do some people have to suffer awful illnesses or tragedies in life? Why do some people clearly have healthier bodies, greater longevity, or simply better luck?

Whether expected or not, an ailment and its consequences do more than alter our lives, whether short term or long. Illness can also be educational, though not the type of instruction that any of us would ever sign up for.

We most easily feel joy when we are healthy, or healthy enough; when we get to do what we like to do, or live the way we want to live. But this is simply not how we get to live all of the time. We become more aware of good health, and more appreciative of it, when we have experienced its absence. This implies somehow that without illness or injury, we would not be maximizing our lives when we do have the capacity.

It is also unclear for whom this wisdom may be intended: the ill may value good health more than ever, less likely to take it for granted if they regain it, but sick folks are sometimes too overwhelmed by their condition to wax philosophical. Most do their best just to hang on and try to get better. One could then wonder if illness also serves to bring out the good in others. Without sickness, there would likely be fewer acts of caring and compassion, because those behaviors would not be required so much in life. Think of all of the people throughout time who have dealt with the unpleasantries of disease, to try to help others in need. The illness of others has motivated caretakers, researchers, and healers, allowing those people to shine through their work.

So, it may not seem like much of a silver lining, but sickness certainly helps us appreciate and value good health, encouraging us to live our own lives well, and to try to help others in need. In the process, that understanding challenges us to respect the mystery and uncertainty of life. Illness therefore may not just be inevitable biologically; perhaps, to some degree, it is a more necessary component of existence than we may realize, teaching us valuable lessons in the process.

Don't get me wrong: given the choice between being wise and enlightened through dealing with illness, or blissfully ignorant and carefree while enjoying good health, I'd choose the latter every time, no question. I imagine that most sane people would. The point, however, is that we do not always get to choose.

Fortunately, we who enjoy good health have the capacity to enhance our own lives while we are still healthy, whether through our own experiences and understanding, or through compassion and empathy, learning from the journeys and burdens of others. Doctors and other health care workers disproportionately see the sickest and least fortunate everyday through our work, and there is a lot to learn from that opportunity and privilege. And yes, it is definitely a privilege.

Again, I'm grateful for every day that I'm on my side of the x-rays. May we all be grateful for what we have, because we will not have it forever.

Whether you see this life as a stepping stone, a trial, a building block, or the only shot that you'll ever get, it's all yours. Make it count.

CROSSING THE BOUNDARY

One afternoon I read a CT scan of a particularly unfortunate woman. She had colon cancer and was only in her early thirties. The tumor in her large intestine had been removed, but after several months she developed new abdominal distension and pain. Her CT scan showed signs of recurrent tumor, as well as fluid accumulation in her pelvis. I called her oncologist and broke the news.

The young woman was then scheduled to have the pelvic fluid drained under CT guidance at the hospital. I was on duty that day. Meeting her the morning of her drainage procedure, I immediately noticed not only her youth but also how nice she was.

"I just finished reviewing your films a few minutes ago," I began. "In fact, I was the one who read your CT the day you had it. Did your oncologist explain what it showed?"

"Yes. She mentioned a new fluid pocket down low, where I've been having pain."

I must have gestured that I would elaborate on her scan's abnormalities, but she continued speaking before I got my next words out.

"Before we go any further," she stated, "there's something that I need to explain. My husband and I are believers."

Caught off guard, I thought I knew what she was implying, but wanted to be sure. She explained without my having to ask a single question.

"We've prayed a great deal, and have family and friends at church praying for me as well. We try not to use the 'C' word, but as far as I'm concerned, my body is cancer free."

She remained pleasant. She looked calm and rational on the surface, but I knew that she was completely wrong about the state of her internal organs. I did not point out that her self-perception did not match her CT scan. I feared that she might forego potentially beneficial treatment options in her denial. My own concern must have been perceptible, because she continued speaking and put me at ease again.

"Now, I'm doing everything the doctors are telling me to—the surgery, the chemotherapy, all of it. But this is what I feel, and what I need to believe to get through this."

"Fair enough," I replied, relieved that I could better understand her outlook, and could respect her regardless. Her approach was different than most people's, but that did not make it wrong. She was not at all accurate about being cancer free, but on some level she knew that, even if she would not outwardly admit it.

We proceeded to go over the steps of her CT drainage. She signed the standard consent form for the procedure, put the pen down on the clipboard, and smiled at me again. "I've got faith," she said, "and I'm putting it in your hands today."

I left the patient in the waiting area for a few minutes until she was called into the CT scanner. As I entered the scanner room where the procedure would take place, I noticed Tara the CT tech positioning the patient on the table. Both were young women, intelligent, friendly, and pretty. One was healthy and in the prime of her life, helping the other whose external youth and attractiveness concealed her bodily illness for the time being.

Tara scanned the woman's pelvis, and I used the images to decide where best to insert the needle. "We know just where to go," I reassured, drawing an "X" on the skin of her lower abdomen with a magic marker. "We'll get started now."

"Before you do," she asked, "could I say a prayer first?"

"Of course," I answered. I had seen many patients over the years briefly lower their heads in silent meditation, never needing to ask permission.

It turned out that this woman's prayer was neither silent nor brief. I was standing on one side of the table, and Tara the CT tech was standing on the other. Lying between us, the patient extended both of her arms with her hands open, gesturing that we each hold one hand while she prayed aloud. Standing across from me, Tara grabbed the patient's left hand, and I placed mine in her right so that the sick woman could begin.

I felt a little uncomfortable at first. Despite a natural interest in humanity and spirituality, outward prayer to me is still a somewhat personal matter, particularly at work. I have never believed that my own religious views or questions are the business of the patients I treat. Being aware of patients' beliefs may occasionally be medically relevant, if the information may help tailor treatment to their needs. However, being asked to participate in her prayer was unusual, and it made me feel a bit awkward. Like most doctors I know, I try to treat everybody with the same dignity and concern, from the atheist to the evangelical of all faiths, without openly bringing my own religion to the equation. When I reached for this woman's hand, I feared that my religious privacy and anonymity might somehow be compromised. The woman, her health, and her faith should be center stage; I only wanted to play a supporting role.

The young patient surprised me yet again. After Tara and I bowed our heads, the patient began her spoken prayer. I could tell she was going to talk longer than most strangers would normally pray aloud, and I braced myself for what I hoped would not feel awkward or insincere. On the contrary, the woman was poised and graceful in her spoken words. The more she talked, the more I found myself relaxing, understanding that the prayer was not about me, other than her expressing thanks for what I might be able to do for her.

"Dear Lord," she began, "I first want to thank you for all of your grace. Thank you so much for guiding these people in their care for me. Thank you for all of this amazing technology and for all of the opportunities you have provided in helping medical care advance so far. It's just so amazing to think of what these people can do with what you've provided, and so amazing to think of all of their education and training that has allowed them to be able to help me and so many others. Thank you for their talents and intelligence and caring as they use your gifts in their work, today and every day."

If her goal was to win compassion through flattery, she

had already succeeded. Her compliments, whether deserved or just hopeful, made me feel capable but humble, able but not overconfident. Her trust was reassuring. I could not imagine letting her down.

Had she stopped right there, I would already have never forgotten her, but she did not stop.

"I pray that your hands will guide theirs in their efforts to help continue to cure me of this disease," she continued. "I ask that you guide us all here so that everything goes smoothly. It really is just incredible, as all of your blessings are, and we all thank you for the glory that you provide. Thank you so much for all of your help in my recovery."

I was still impressed with her gratitude and sincerity. Her denial of the CT scan findings was still foreign to me, but it did not matter anymore. She was not truly delusional; she simply had to believe that she would be healed. She was positive, gracious, and genuine. She approached her disease with the medical understanding that she could not outwardly admit, and with the religious conviction to which she clung in her time of need.

"As always," she concluded, "thank you for the love of my family and friends, for my faith in you, for the support of my church, and for all who seek to serve you and perform your work. We continue to ask for your guidance and understanding as we pray to you, Lord. Thank you, Jesus, my Savior, for all that you do always, for all of your blessings. Thank you for your help and love and for guiding me through this ordeal. In your name we pray, Lord, Jesus Christ. Amen."

"Amen," Tara across from me replied softly, nodding her head once, then raising up from her bowed position. I wondered how much her reply was from the heart, or how much was for the benefit of the patient, but never was sure that it would be appropriate to ask.

"Amen," I echoed, afraid of waiting any longer.

The patient and her prayer left me feeling surprisingly comfortable. I had just been asked not only to witness, but also to participate in her religious practice. That experience might have been unsettling in another context. Yet, the gratitude and peace that she emitted left me feeling tranquil, clearly focused, and somehow empowered. Some might wonder if the prayer's power might have resulted from a higher intervention. Not qualified to confirm with any certainty, I can say that the three of us present felt the confidence and strength to perform the task at hand. We were helping her, and she was helping us to help her, without anyone assuming or forcing any beliefs on the other people. She may have needed to be overtly religious, but in essence only asked that we be supportive by allowing her the outward expression.

The drainage went reasonably well, but not ideally. We did get some fluid out, but not as much as I had hoped. The fluid was walled off and compartmentalized, like liquid in a sponge. One needle stick could not drain it all. A second puncture removed a little more, but the cancerous fluid was too complex, the drainage too challenging. Repeated punctures would be even less beneficial. We stopped after getting what we readily could. Her pain was partly relieved, but not so much as I wish we could have provided. Still, she understood that we did the best we could, and thanked us again before departing.

She did return for a follow up CT scan several weeks later, but on a day when I was working at another office in the practice. I never met her again. About two months after the day we met, I saw her obituary in the newspaper.

Note: an earlier version of this story was published as "My Patient's Faith", *UUWorld* Vol. XXV No. 2, Summer 2011.

RELATIVE RISK

A serious injury at any age can be devastating. But when tragedy strikes someone young in the physical prime of life, the consequences are particularly horrifying—even when such events can provide insight and lessons for us all.

The body is a wonder which never ceases to amaze in its intricate structure. Our healthy bodies allow us to experience all the elements that compose our lives; they give us motion and thought, purpose, accomplishment, and joy. When serious illness or injury is revealed with x-rays, the pictures are ominous, foreshadowing limitations and challenges which could be too great to bear if not for the resilience and adaptation of the human spirit.

Such was the case one evening at the hospital, when a young woman in surgical residency came to review a teenage boy's spinal x-ray with me.

"This looks horrible," I told her. "What happened to him?"

"Motocross accident," she said, shaking her head. "He's only fifteen. He's got a total sensory and motor deficit from the waist down. They're still assessing him in the emergency room, but he's coming over here shortly for a CT scan. We'll also want an MRI of his spine tonight."

"Absolutely." The scans would be done, but the one x-ray view of the teenager's thoracic spine already revealed plenty. A vertebra in his mid back was crushed, markedly disrupting his spinal alignment. At the fracture, his spine had separated, pulling his spinal cord too far in the wrong direction. Bone fragments had broken off and lodged within the canal where his spinal cord should have been, pressing upon his probably severed cord. Bleeding would further compress this delicate central nervous tissue.

"Is he going to surgery?" I asked her.

"Probably, after his scans. We've still got to rule out any abdominal injury before the neurosurgeons take him to the operating room."

Moments later the youth was brought to the CT scanner.

"Everybody ready, on the count of three," the surgery resident said, as other residents and x-ray technologists carefully slid the boy on a backboard from the CT table onto a stretcher.

"My back hurts," he cried, "it hurts!" Yet even more frightening to him, and more concerning to the rest of us, was the absence of pain, or any other sensation, or any ability to move, below that level.

"I can't feel my legs!" he cried repeatedly. "Oh, God!"

His family stood weeping outside the door in the hallway, protected from the radiation, but in full range of the emotional devastation.

Unable to offer any encouraging words, I retreated to the dark shadows of my reading room to study his case in detail. By the time I finished interpreting his CT scan, he had been transferred down the hall for the MRI of his spine, before his expected back surgery. An eerie calm briefly replaced the commotion. Soon the neurosurgeons would come to review the boy's scans with me. They would then break the news to the teenager and his family, before doing what they could to try to stabilize his spine.

The CT provided some fracture detail not visible on the initial x-ray, and the MRI showed his spinal cord, which was completely severed. Short of a future scientific miracle, he would be paralyzed from the waist down for the rest of his life.

Hours before he had enjoyed a healthy, perfectly functioning body—the picture of youth, promise and potential, nearly matured to the human ideal. That ideal was trashed forever in an unfortunate, indelible instant, in an activity considered optional at best, reckless by many.

Many of us are drawn to fitness exercises that provide a sense of strength and well-being, and to other physical activities that offer sensations of thrill. Motocross is something I have no direct experience with, having only seen it on brief occasion while changing television channels. Youngsters on dirt bikes, in colorful outfits with helmets and goggles, flying through the air, doing tricks; landing precariously, churning up clods of earth with thickly treaded tires, wheels spinning, motors roaring; boys hanging onto handle bars, trying to steady themselves, trying not to fall off, or tip over, or get hurt; or, perhaps believing, at that seemingly invincible age, that true harm will not happen to them.

Now that activity, and the devastating injury that resulted, would prevent him from doing many of the seemingly simplest tasks that most of us take for granted daily. Unless scientists discover a safe way to regenerate healthy central nervous tissue within this young man's lifetime, his chances of ever walking again are abysmal. He will be forever restricted to a wheelchair or bed, limited in motion and feeling.

After getting through the initial physical and psychological adjustment periods, he will be predisposed to other complications common with paralysis, like infections and skin ulcers. He may be incontinent, or have to catheterize every time he needs to empty his bladder. All of these limitations could impact his longevity, his career options, and his personal relationships. At age fifteen, he also may have experienced his last orgasm, and may have never felt the joy of sharing one with another human being. He will be limited in where he can go, and in what he can do, for the rest of his life.

We all seek excitement at times, new thrills that make life more appealing, more fun, more challenging and memorable. Most of us also admit that we have done risky things at times, and might have had an equally tragic outcome, had we not been lucky enough to surface unscathed. How unbelievably fortunate most of us are to have avoided similar fates, when we may have at one time or another engaged in risky activities.

I felt grateful to walk to my car late that night, grateful to walk at all. I was thankful to have gone to the pool to swim laps before work that evening. I remembered the thrill of diving into the cool water, of pulling myself along with smooth, coordinated movements, to feel agile and unrestricted; to glide, to feel powerful, to move freely. I was grateful to drive home uneventfully, and to arrive home safely; grateful to be able to climb the stairs and crawl into bed. Nevertheless, the weight of that teenager's case kept me from sleeping peacefully that night.

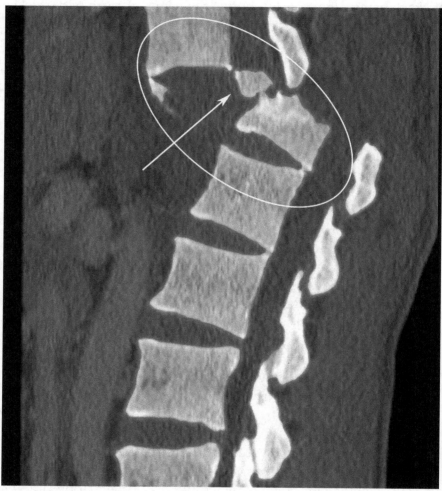

Paralysis from spinal cord injury post vertebral fracture and displacement

CT scan lateral projection showing a vertebral fracture with displacement (circled). A large bone fragment (arrow) has migrated into the spinal canal, compressing and disrupting the spinal cord. —Image courtesy of Brian Choi, MD

The very next morning the newspaper featured an article about a man close to my age. He had suffered a spinal cord injury as a youth and, like the youngster at the hospital the night before, had been paralyzed from the waist down. The man had also become an accomplished long-distance swimmer, years after his injury.

He had only his upper body with which to propel himself through the water, but he had trained to become a better swimmer than most people who are in perfect health. He also had a successful career, and from all indications, a meaningful life. He never lost his mind, his creativity, or his imagination. Evidently he also kept his determination.

I then remembered other people I have known who lived much of their lives in wheelchairs, including a police chief; an accomplished artist; a young woman who went on to marry and have a family; and two doctors with whom I have worked. These individuals did not even come to mind immediately, because when I think of them, I first think of the people—not their wheelchairs.

Picturing the teenager's broken back and torn spinal cord, I still shuddered for him in his condition, and fear that he may suffer so many of the other complications that result from paralysis. And yet, when thinking of others who adapt to survive the disabilities that impact their lives, I hope and pray that his injury does not extinguish the spark, or ironically, the appreciation that even a very limited physical existence can provide. Despite his obvious bodily restrictions, some of the factors that define a life as meaningful and worthwhile may still be within his power.

Yo-Yo

She worked as an x-ray tech at one of the practice's busiest offices. She was tall and fair, with glasses and very short red hair. A mother in her forties, she had a youthful exuberance, combined with a pleasant calmness. She was never loud, but often smiled. I never heard her complain. Her name was Yolanda, but people sometimes called her "Yo-Yo."

She is the only woman over forty that I ever saw post pictures of young male celebrities on a bulletin board at work. Her taste in men, at least from the magazine pictures she displayed, appeared to be only slightly more mature than that of the average teenage girl. She avoided almost all vegetables like a finicky child, ordering her lunchtime sandwiches on white bread, with no lettuce or tomato. She was funny and well-liked by the other staff members at work, befriending people considerably younger and older than she.

She did not make a drastic impression on me initially. I thought of her as a nice, likeable, and competent person who was a pleasure to work with, but it took some time to get to know her more closely. Without wearing emotions on her sleeve or being overly revealing about her personal life, she seemed happy to come to work, do a good job, and mingle with her co-workers.

Yet she surprised me one morning when I came to work. Instead of wearing the usual cotton scrubs and standing in the x-ray work area, she was seated in the room for patients, next to the CT scanner, wearing a light blue gown. A co-worker was placing an IV into Yo-Yo's forearm.

"Yolanda," I said with amazement. "What are you doing having a CT scan? Are you feeling okay?"

"I feel fine," she replied. "I've had breast cancer, and am

just getting a follow-up study to see how it's doing on this chemotherapy."

"I didn't even know you were sick," I said. Yolanda was never shy about having me check her difficult x-ray cases, but she had never mentioned her own illness to me.

"I don't think of myself as sick," she responded. "I know I have lesions in my liver, but I feel fine. This chemo's not bad, so it's really not bothering me right now."

It was astounding to hear her reveal that she not only had cancer, but metastatic cancer. I went about my work, later learning from other co-workers who knew her better that she had been dealing with cancer for some time. She was not keeping it a secret, but she did not dwell on it either. She was calm and determined to keep going with a business-as-usual approach, seemingly cool on the exterior, despite what her body looked like on the inside.

I read her CT scan later that morning, comparing the images to her prior studies. By the time I was reading her new CT films, she had already had her IV pulled, changed from the blue gown to her work clothes, and was busy taking x-rays of other patients.

I would read several of her x-ray studies over the next couple of years. Sometimes a new chemotherapy regimen would make the liver metastases smaller, at least for a while. She had a CT of her head once when she was having headaches, and the study fortunately revealed that no tumor had spread to her brain. Another time, I scanned her liver by ultrasound when a blood test showed a high level of bilirubin, a component of liver bile. Her doctor knew this could be a side effect of her chemotherapy, but wanted to make sure her bile ducts were not blocked by tumor in her liver. I saw no blockage of her bile ducts, but the degree of tumor involvement within her liver was striking. Her liver looked significantly worse than it had on a CT scan only a few months before. Yo-Yo went back to work that day, looking like her usual self on the job.

Other than these times when our relationship required my medical input, she kept the same sense of humor, interests, topics of conversation, and energy level. Always professional and respectful with patients, in the break room she proudly continued to display an occasional new magazine photograph of the latest male Hollywood heartthrob who struck her fancy. She also played practical jokes. One day in the office, a young, good-looking male x-ray tech was spending extra time talking with an attractive young woman after taking her x-ray. He clearly remained within his professional bounds, yet he was engaged in a mild flirtation with the equally interested patient. Yo-Yo realized that their conversation was several minutes beyond the x-ray instruction of "hold still and don't breathe," and she could not resist sticking her head through the door. In a very audible voice she exclaimed, "Jason, your wife just called. You have to pick up the kids at day care after work today." Jason, single and childless, was too caught off guard to reply. The patient gave him a look and left the office.

Months passed, and Yo-Yo kept us updated after visits with her oncologist, and after her follow-up CT scans. We all knew that her long-term prognosis was not good, but Yo-Yo's casual manner kept the topic from being depressing. She offered new information when she had something to share, and people listened and asked questions with genuine interest and concern. Otherwise, we simply talked about other things. She continued to work hard in the busy x-ray office, keeping up with people younger and healthier than herself.

I told her once that I admired her stamina and positive thinking.

"I just like feeling healthy and normal," she replied. "I find that if I stay busy and keep working, I feel more like a normal person." I nodded with approval, and admiration, but only partial understanding. For years I have believed that people with a minor illness, such as a common cold, may feel more like their normal selves if they continue their regular routines, including light exercise, and ignore the ailment until it passes. However, I could not compare a life's worth of common colds to the illness that she was battling. Her perseverance was inspiring and very admirable. It would have been completely understandable and justifiable for her to work less, spending more time with loved ones or pursuing other interests while she could. She may have been heading in that direction eventually, but opted instead to show up at the office daily, punch in on the time clock, and work hard, for considerably less money than I make.

More months passed, and Yo-Yo took thousands of more x-rays on the job, between jokes with co-workers. One day she came into my office with no x-ray in hand, and hesitantly began posing a question. Seeing her tentative nature, I assumed she would be asking my medical opinion about one of her latest treatments. She surprised me by expressing that she was slightly concerned that she had never seen a picture of my significant other. She explained that it was important to her that both parties in a couple be similar in physical attractiveness, and she inadvertently complimented me by wanting to make sure that I was adequately matched. This was in the days before smart phones and social media accounts, so I told her that I would gladly bring a picture to work for her to inspect.

Given that she was dealing with her ongoing illness, plus the pressures of full-time work, her marriage and children, I thought it peculiar but comical that she could put aside anxieties about her own mortality in order to concern herself with the physical appeal of my mate at that time. I did indeed bring a suitable photograph, which Yo-Yo reviewed. She nodded with approval and seemed satisfied.

"I guess you would also feel reassured to hear that we are compatible in many ways, and that we try to be respectful and supportive of each other?" I teased.

"Oh no," she countered in complete seriousness. "I just wanted to make sure that you both look good together. That's important to me."

Undoubtedly she had her private moments, but she did not easily reveal them at work. Whenever she suffered a setback in her physical condition, she rebounded quickly. A complication might arise from a new chemotherapy, but she would get past the inconvenience, put it behind her as best as she could, and be back on the job soon, smiling and working as productively as always.

I still teased her about her nearly child-like distaste for vegetables, but granted that after all she had been through, she could feel entitled to indulge in, or abstain from, whatever she wanted.

As time progressed, symptoms appeared that were harder to ignore. Her cycle of ailments and temporary improvements was accelerating, gradually spinning toward a lesser degree of control. Yo-Yo struggled to bounce back, but the gravity of her illness kept pulling her down for increasingly heavier and longer periods. Hospitalizations became more frequent. Fluid began to accumulate in her abdomen, requiring drainage by ultrasound guidance. She must have been privately distressed that she was beginning to spiral downward, but she at least found a small delight in winning the office college basketball pool while recovering from another physical setback. Yo-Yo kept trying and snapped back again, recuperating at home for alarmingly short periods of time before coming back to work. She would be discharged from her latest stay at the hospital, rest only a few days, and then return to work to serve patients with physical problems less severe than her own. Still, she never complained. Only toward the end of her working days did she have no choice but to acknowledge physical pain, before reluctantly taking some afternoons off to go home and rest. We watched her put up one of the most impressive fights imaginable, refusing to be conquered for as long as possible.

One day when I was working at the hospital, I got a call from one of the other x-ray technologists at the office, where Yo-Yo was no longer working. "Yolanda called this morning," she said. "The doctors have decided that the chemo is doing more harm than good, and they've recommended that she stop receiving any further treatment. They're arranging hospice care."

"I'm really sorry to hear that."

"I know, we all are, but I knew you'd want an update. She asked about you. She said that the card you sent her recently did her more good than a round of chemo. It meant so much to her that she felt like writing you a thank-you note."

"She does not have to formally thank me for a card," I said.

"I know," she replied, "but you know how she is. Can you believe that she was telling us this morning not to worry about her getting hospice, and that she's not going down without a fight? I genuinely think she's worried about us and our reactions to the news of her hospice care."

We agreed to pay her a visit soon, after Yo-Yo got settled into a new routine with relatives arriving from out of town. However, the events that followed in the next few days were anything but routine.

Most people, at least occasionally, talk about feeling tired or overextended, taking for granted the level of health that we have. Yo-Yo would put most people to shame. Before I open my mouth at times to express fatigue from work, I hope that I remember Yo-Yo's example. She gracefully moved along her erratic and unpredictable physical course in a manner that would impress anyone who took notice. I do not ever expect to meet anyone with such a remarkable work ethic, stamina, or determination to outdo an illness that literally zaps the life out of people. I certainly hope that her strengths and character endured to the end.

How ironic that one person's experience with cancer could somehow be partly refreshing to everyone who knew her. Her personal example on the outside was everything that her body could not be on the inside. Still, when I think of her humor, her positive attitude, and her persistence, I am somehow left remembering one of the healthiest people I have ever known.

SELF DISCOVERY

The first time our instructor walked into the hospital conference room, he reminded me of a middle-aged Malibu Ken doll—blond, tan, blue-eyed, and preppy, but with a few lines on his face, and the slightest paunch under his green surgical scrub top. As soon as he spoke in his educated but clearly Southern drawl, his California looks ceded to his Carolina roots. "I don't know if y'all drew the short stick or the long, but I'll be your instructor for this seminar on social and cultural issues in medicine. I've got colleagues also teaching small groups like this, and they're just planning to sit around and discuss treating patients. That's fine, but I have a different philosophy. I can't teach you nearly so much by just talking about patients as I can by having you actually meet some."

He sat up straight in his chair, buttoned his long, white coat, then leaned forward and gazed at the ten of us medical students seated at the table, newly enrolled in August of 1988. "Even though you all are just getting started in your training, it's never too soon to work on mastering the art of patient interaction. It can make or break you—I've seen both happen to colleagues. I want each and every one of you to understand that how well you understand patients, and how well they understand you, are strengths that cannot be overemphasized."

Unsure what to make of his enthusiasm, we nodded while he kept talking. "I'm planning to bring a patient to class each week for you all to interview, as a group. After each session, do some research on the symptoms and see if you can't come up with some likely diagnoses to report back."

He was a board certified urologist and medical professor.

222

We were brand new students just learning the basics of human anatomy and physiology, intimidated by his expectations. He read the unspoken fear on our faces. "An accurate diagnosis isn't the most important thing at this point. I know you don't know much medicine yet, but you're here to learn. Just show me your thought process." He smiled. "It'll be fun."

"Now, if you're going to talk to patients, they need to look at you as student doctors. When we meet in this class each week from now on for the rest of the semester, I want you to come wearing white coats. You will need to buy them eventually for your hospital rotations, so go ahead and get one now in order to look professional. You young men wear a necktie, and I'm sure the women in the class will look appropriate as well. Today you'll be OK as you are, because the patient is someone I work with."

A few minutes later, a young, lean man with dark curly hair and a moustache walked in and said hello. He looked healthy.

"Have a seat at the end of the table," our professor invited. "Mr. Johnson here is one of the secretaries in the hospital, on the ward where most of the urology patients stay, so we know each other. It gets kind of hectic and stressful around here sometimes." The young man nodded in agreement with the professor. "When he asked earlier today if he could speak with me about a medical issue, I told him I needed someone for this class, and he politely agreed to come and talk with you. Mr. Johnson, these students would like to ask a few questions."

We took turns asking him what symptoms he was having, for how long, if he was taking any medicine, what his family history was, and so on. He was polite, but the answers were not elucidating— mild abdominal pain, occasional diarrhea or constipation, no visible bleeding. We had no idea what was wrong with him.

Two things happened by the next class the following week: one student found a textbook description of irritable bowel syndrome that might fit the man's symptoms; and another classmate saw the young patient in a local bar a few days later and said hello. The man seemed slightly embarrassed, confessing that he was not really sick but had been pretending in order that we had a patient to interview that day.

"So," our classmate said before our professor arrived for the second session, "we may be getting actors each week. Don't let on that we know."

The teacher walked in, still wearing surgical scrubs, with disposable paper covers still on his shoes from the operating room. A red line indented his forehead where his surgical cap had just been untied. He sat down, ran his fingers through his blond bangs, and buttoned his loose white coat.

"It's been quite a day," he began. "I saw forty patients in clinic before noon, then I was in the O.R. until just a minute ago. That's the way you have to do it most days, if you're going to survive in this business. Anyway, the group style interview last week was OK, but I think it will be easier for the patients to focus if you all take turns each week being the primary interviewer. The rest of the class can observe, then ask questions at the end. Any volunteers for today?"

No one moved, so after a brief but uncomfortable pause, I raised my hand.

"Good. She'll be here shortly. Well, any thoughts on the patient last week?"

We concealed that we thought it was all an act, while one student presented his consideration of irritable bowel syndrome. The teacher listened but said nothing.

Suddenly a moving shadow hit the doorway from the corridor outside. Up rolled an old woman in a wheelchair, pushed by a young black orderly. The old lady wore only a light blue hospital gown, with a blanket across her lap. A bag of clear fluid was hanging on a metal pole attached to the wheelchair, slowly dripping into an IV in her forearm. Clipped to the side of the chair was a catheter bag filled with blood-tinged urine. Wide-eyed, the student who had seen the previous young male patient at the bar looked at me. "Dude," I whispered, "this is no act."

I was twenty-three years old, and although I had visited people in hospitals before, I was still unaccustomed to seeing people in that condition. I felt slightly unsure how to begin the interview. Everyone was watching though, so I decided that it should not be too different than talking to one's grandmother. I introduced myself and began asking questions. The woman was sweet, appreciative, kind, and forthcoming. Once we got started, the conversation flowed smoothly, illustrating that when you ask people about themselves in a caring way, they usually carry the conversation, revealing what you need to know in the midst of what they convey.

Toward the end of the interview, our professor asked the woman a question. "Ma'am, do you remember the first time we met at my office?"

"I certainly do," she smiled.

"Just out of curiosity," he inquired, "how long do you remember my talking with you that first visit?"

"I'd say an hour." We stared at her in silence, collectively doubting that he could have spent so long with one patient, if he just saw forty patients in one morning. She noticed our staring, evidently interpreting our disbelief. "Well, I don't know, it was at least a half-hour."

After the interview I thanked her and wished her luck. She reached out, grabbed my arms, and thanked me as sincerely as I could ever recall having been thanked. The only thing we did for her was show her that we cared, and it was all she required of us that day.

After she was wheeled back to her hospital room, the doctor confessed that their first visit had lasted twelve minutes. "I had the nurse knock on the door after ten minutes, in order for me to get to the next patient waiting. One important way to make people think that you've spent more time with them than you actually may have is to sit down in front of them, and look at them at eye level. As important as it is to be thorough with patients and listen well, you'll never make it if you can't keep them moving."

It seemed oddly manipulative, but this woman greatly respected him and was grateful for the care he provided. Her satisfaction helped us realize that he was not being truly deceptive. He had only a finite time to allot any given patient, and he wanted the experience maximized for each one.

"All right, good job for your first interview," he said. "Any questions before next week?"

"Yes," one woman in the class replied. "What's the answer with the man from last week?"

"Oh—he's gay, and he was worried if he needed to be tested for AIDS." That fact was no surprise in itself, but the ten of us students had not gotten that information in over thirty minutes of joint interview, yet the young man had volunteered it immediately to our professor, whom he trusted.

The series of patient interviews and seminars over the semester remained quite educational, particularly since most of us students had no previous clinical experience. Although we had a lot to learn over the upcoming years, we did break the ice in learning to feel comfortable talking to patients, sometimes having to ask awkward or intimate questions.

The young medical professor was a good role model for several reasons. Most importantly, he was very enthusiastic about his work. "Each patient is unique," he explained. "Don't forget that. Just when you think that things are becoming routine or predictable, a new twist in a case will throw a wrench into the familiarity. Don't let that make you uncomfortable—that's just one of the things that helps keep this field so exciting."

He did seem a bit intense, revealing to our seminar group that he had voluntarily retaken the national medical board examination a second time only the year before. "I passed it the first time back when I needed to—but as a teacher training students and residents, I just wanted to see what kinds of questions they're asking these days." Of course it might have looked poorly if a board-certified surgical instructor had not performed as well on the examination as he once had as a medical student, so he studied thoroughly for months before the unnecessary repeat exam, making sure that his score would be at least as strong as the first time around. I could picture his children, wondering why their dad might be too busy to play, choosing to spend hours studying for a test he did not have to take.

As intense as his fervor for medicine was, he definitely had a sense of humor, even if the humor we saw in class was often of a medical nature. Once he explained the different intensive care units at the hospital: "There's the Pediatric Intensive Care Unit," he began, "known as the PICU, or *pick-you*. There's the surgical intensive care unit, known as the SICU, or the 'sick-you'. The Neonatal Intensive Care Unit, or NICU, is called the 'nick-you'. And then there's the Follow Up Care Unit," he winked.

Among his patients with urinary troubles, a large percentage included older men with difficulty urinating due to an enlarged prostate. These men would often ask the urologist what causes prostate enlargement. At the time, the answer was that nobody really knew for sure. Yet when posed with the question, the doctor would look at these men directly and reply, "Too much sex and not enough alcohol," with a twinkle in his eye.

Despite emphasizing the importance of speed and efficiency in a medical practice, he also stressed that these goals cannot compromise accuracy. "Your greatest responsibility is to the patient you're treating. Don't ever forget that, lest you find yourself sitting in front of twelve strangers."

Later that semester, one of the class requirements was that students have an actual hospital patient interview videotaped, with the taped interview reviewed by the class for constructive criticism. "Don't forget to look professional. I once saw a surgical resident in the hospital on a Saturday, wearing sweatpants while interviewing a newly admitted patient. Don't ever let me catch you doing that. At least go put on some surgical scrubs, if you're not wearing a presentable outfit at the time. And don't forget that white coat."

The day came when it was time to review my videotaped interview. Days before I had gone to the hospital, neatly dressed in my short white coat, and met a small, middle-aged black woman who had consented to the taped dialogue. She had endured more health problems than most women her age, particularly rheumatoid arthritis, but also high blood pressure, diabetes, and kidney trouble. Never having finished high school, she had worked doing laundry until her joint pain made employment difficult. She lived nearby with a grown son. She was nice, quiet and soft-spoken, but not always forthcoming with information. Many of her answers were brief, leaving me to wonder if I was doing more of the talking than perhaps I should.

"Have you ever had any trouble with your heart?" I asked midway into the interview.

"No," she shook her head. Ten minutes later, in the midst of discussing other systems of her body, she volunteered, "I had bypass surgery."

"You had bypass surgery? For your heart?" She nodded. I realized that patients sometimes need to communicate at their own speed or comfort level. Just attempting to take a history does not mean that all pertinent information has been revealed.

Later in the interview I asked her about her arthritis, which had distorted the shape of her ankles and wrists. "Are you still able to function in your usual manner?" I asked. She looked at me blankly and said nothing. I rephrased: "Can you still work around the house?"

"Yes," she said, reminding me that the more I speak the patients' language, the more they'll communicate to me.

The rest of the taped interview went smoothly. The class watched the tape together, the whole discussion with the woman lasting about ten minutes.

"Cullen, that was good. Now you obviously can be articulate, which is fine, but I guarantee you lost her when you asked her whether or not she could function in her usual manner." I smiled in agreement. "Fortunately, you recognized that and rebounded by bringing the conversation back to a level she was comfortable with, which is key."

I was pleased, and relieved. However, I could barely contain myself from laughing out loud with his last bit of constructive criticism. "You may have noticed that the back of your white coat was ever so slightly raised above your shoulders when you sat down," he explained. "Just as a point of style, always be sure to sit on the tail of your coat, so it stays more snug across your back and shoulders in the seated position." My classmates and I laughed about this after class, likening his advice to that given by the character of a superficial anchorman in a scene from the movie "Broadcast News."

The doctor enjoyed telling us of the hard work that had gone into accomplishing his goals. He almost boasted that he could see eighty patients in one clinic day. He was proud of mastering the fatigue of his surgical residency, when he spent every other night at the hospital, getting very little sleep. He belittled the fact that surgical residencies had changed in hospital call requirements to every third night for many rotations. "Those of us who did every other night call in the hospital just guffaw at every third night call. They work one night, sleep the second, and can actually *read* the third evening!"

Still relatively new to medical school, I did not think it unreasonable that anybody would actually have one free night at home out of three, when not so exhausted as to immediately collapse from treating patients the night before. If all surgical residents needed to have that degree of stamina, plus a little cockiness, I thought it wise to consider another field of specialty.

The doctor was equally proud of his wife, whom he praised several times. A successful academic ear, nose, and throat specialist at the same university, she had earned very good grades as a medical student, and had put herself through school by taking extra jobs, incurring minimal debt. Her work ethic and dedication matched his, and he glowed when he spoke of her. He may have been a little proud, but he was more humbly proud of her.

Despite his work intensity, a slight tone of accomplishment, and even an occasionally superficial side to some of his advice, he taught our small group a great deal. I did not want to be exactly like him, but I definitely liked, respected, and admired him.

At the end of the semester, he revealed that he and his wife would be leaving the medical school faculty. They had decided to move to a different town, and both would go into private practice. Finishing our last class on a warm spring day, we thanked him for his advice and guidance, and wished him well in his new professional endeavor.

A short while after the physician couple did indeed resign their faculty positions and move to their new locale, we learned of a most unusual turn of events. The doctor purchased an ultrasound machine for his new urology office, in order to have some of his patients' studies performed on site. When the machine arrived, he plugged it in and turned it on in order to try it out. Before scanning a single patient, he tested the machine by scanning his own kidneys. On one of them he found a tumor.

As a urologist who specialized in operating on kidneys and the urinary tract, he knew that the tumor was likely cancerous, as it turned out to be. It had been there the whole time he taught our class, only no one knew, least of all himself. He had the kidney removed, but the cancer had already spread to some lymph nodes. His odds of surviving were quite poor.

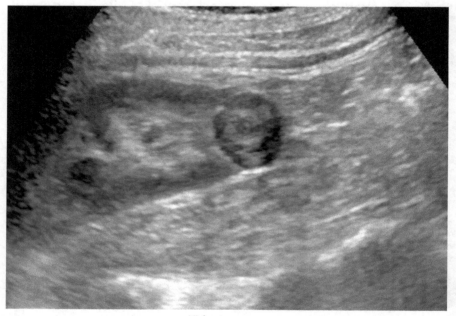

Kidney cancer
Ultrasound of a solid mass in a kidney, renal cell carcinoma.

We wrote cards to him while he underwent experimental chemotherapy that left him feeling very sick. Ultimately he would succumb to a disease that he had himself successfully treated in many other patients, people who had been lucky enough to have their cancers discovered at earlier, curable stages.

By literally looking into himself on a whim, he discovered the cause of his own mortality. His recently made plans were drastically changed. Rather than being more in charge of his professional work in a new private practice, he would now have to surrender himself to the hands of others, who would treat him as well as they knew how. Rather than being more in control of his life, he had to surrender to a destiny he could not control. He would have to adjust his style to maximize the time, impact, and experiences he had remaining. His literal self-discovery by imaging would require a greater degree of metaphorical discovery through introspection and reflection, as he would figuratively look within for the rest of his remaining life.

When doctors read images, we do feel sorry for people in whom we find serious abnormalities, even when the patient is unknown to us, as is usually the case with modern imaging. We try to remain objective, but in some sense, we can still feel the weight and potential consequences of an ominous discovery. If the person imaged happens to be someone we know, and we find something bad, then the gravity of the diagnosis usually feels even more intense and personal. In his case, the discovery was of the ultimate ominous nature: reading a study with a fatal disease, knowing that the body imaged was his own.

IKE

The first week of medical school, our anatomy professor addressed our class in the filled auditorium, speaking into a microphone clipped to his long white lab coat. His hair was thinned, his face pale, and his manner more relaxed than the new and slightly nervous students seated before him. Many of us, in our shorts and backpacks, could still pass for undergraduate students on campus, while our professor looked as if he had been teaching that class for a long time.

"Before we proceed to the dissection labs," he began, "you should be reassured that most people naturally have some reluctance to touch a dead body, not to mention cut on one. Remember, human dissection is a rite of passage that physicians in training have gone through for hundreds of years. I assume that most of you have not worked with human cadavers before, but trust that your intellectual curiosity will quickly provide an adequate comfort level. Let me now review a couple of basic points regarding cutting, so as to perform a neat dissection and not injure yourselves."

He then turned on a bright lightbulb within an overhead projector hovering over a small table at the front of the lecture hall. The small tabletop displayed onto the screen behind him for us to see, larger than life. On the table was a green cotton surgical towel about one square foot in size, draped over an object bulging up from underneath. He lifted the towel and revealed what looked like a segment of a human forearm, cut out between the hand and elbow. As he picked it up in his hands, we could see that it was the size of a child's forearm. Many of us were not convinced that it was genuine.

"Is that real?" a student next to me asked in disbelief.

"I'm not sure," I whispered. "Look at the skin color; it looks like a doll's arm." Other students had come to the same conclusion. A couple classmates even giggled quietly at the absurdity of trying to pass this plastic replica off as human tissue.

"Work cautiously and gently, but pressing firmly enough to make a single clean incision," he demonstrated, cutting into the skin, peeling back the top layer to reveal the plane of tissue beneath.

The silence was palpable. The barely audible nervous chuckling by a couple of students moments ago had stopped, replaced with our collective, ominous realization that the specimen was indeed real, from a child who had at least lost an arm, probably a life.

"We have made available some 3-D models, x-ray and CT studies that you may find helpful in learning anatomy," he continued. "These are only complementary, of course, and cannot take the place of directly visualizing the structures you must learn. Before we conclude here and go to the labs, I remind you all of the special gift that your cadavers have provided. Their bodies were donated for the purpose of your education. Please treat them respectfully."

"One more thing," he said, lightening his tone. "In addition to the gloves provided in the labs, you will find that washing your hands with lime shaving cream is particularly helpful in removing the stench of the formaldehyde preservative."

So began our education in human anatomy, a fundamental of medical training. Every student in the medical field expects to perform cadaver dissection, learning the layout of our internal organs. What I did not expect, by studying one dead man's anatomy, was to gain a greater appreciation for the complexities and composition of life itself.

Our medical school provided one cadaver for every four students. On the first day of anatomy class, we entered the laboratory where we would spend three afternoons a week for several months, slowly dissecting the cadavers according to the outlined lessons. The cadavers were neatly laid face up on metal dissecting tables, sealed in airtight plastic bags with a long zipper down the middle. Our instructors had become accustomed to human dissection years ago, and to completely green beginning students like ourselves, the teachers seemed surprisingly unfazed by their work.

The four students in our group were assigned a large man, who looked as if he had died around age seventy. He was tall and muscular despite his age. His name and history were a mystery to us. The stranger looked at peace lying on the table, while the quartet of new medical students began the process of slowly opening him up and taking his body apart.

One of the two young women in our group spoke nervously. "Since we're starting on his chest, would you all mind if we cover his face?"

"No, no, not at all," we echoed.

"I don't like the thought of him staring out anyway, even if his eyes are closed and he's facing the ceiling," the other young man in the group said.

I agreed. "I know he doesn't feel any pain as a dead man, but it's still weird cutting into him, as if I'm afraid we're going to hurt him somehow."

As our comfort levels increased, our affinity for the cadavers also improved. This is not to imply that the dissection experience itself was ever particularly enjoyable, but rather that we came to appreciate the man on the table, and what he offered us as we learned from him. We were becoming progressively more intimate with his internal composition, and we thought it appropriate that we recognize him as a trusted acquaintance.

"I think we need to give our cadaver a name," I said during the second week. The others agreed, but none of us had a suitable suggestion. Some students in other groups started calling their cadavers old-fashioned names like Gladys or Wilbur. Some chose nicknames based on famous people. We were at a loss.

"There's no rush. We'll think of something that suits him."

After a short period of adjustment, the anatomy lab experience became quite interesting. Once comfortable dissecting our cadavers, most of us often found the exercises to be practical and intriguing. Sometimes the outlined organs were easier to find than others. Other times we wondered why we had to locate and memorize the names of so many smaller parts. Although every part of the body serves some purpose or another, memorizing the names of every small muscle and nerve seemed more for purposes of academic trivia than future practical relevance.

Occasionally students briefly examined other groups' cadavers within the anatomy laboratory. We knew which groups of students had large cadavers, small cadavers, men, or women. Organs might be easier to find in the thinner cadavers, but identifying muscles tended to be easier in the more developed or less emaciated bodies. For educational purposes, it behooved us to compare and contrast the cadaver we knew best with the others in the room, since we would eventually need to recognize organs within patients of all shapes and sizes.

The weeks continued. Despite the relative comfort we had grown into, there were still parts of the body that were generally more emotionally difficult to dissect than others, namely the face, hands, and genitalia. When assigned to dissect these parts of the body, some of us felt squeamish, as if we were beginning the dissection process all over again. Although the rational mind knows that a corpse does not feel pain, it is hard to cut into a sensitive part of the body and not fear hurting that person. We had to force ourselves over the hurdles of apprehension in order to make the first incision into these nearly sacred structures. I believe the difficulty lay in the fact that these particular body parts are external, full of nerve endings, and tend to be the aspects of the body that most outwardly express one's personality. A liver or lung may not look that different from one person to the next, or even when compared to another mammal. In contrast, a person's hands, genitals, and facial features are somehow more special, personal, and undeniably human.

Still, my group was unable to think of a suitable name for our cadaver, until the day we isolated the heart. We noticed that the coronary arteries, which supply blood to the heart muscle, were hard with heavy calcium deposits. We pointed this out to the instructor walking between the tables.

"Yeah, that makes sense in his case," he confirmed. Usually this teacher spoke with a graceful style, impeccably reciting the Latin-based names of the body parts in his African American southern accent. His candor that moment when talking about our cadaver was a departure from his typical demeanor.

"Why do you say that?" we collectively asked, puzzled by his statement.

"Because this guy died by having a heart attack while slapping his wife around," he replied.

We stood back from the table and looked at the embalmed human form with disgust and disappointment. The affinity that we had previously felt for this man was shattered. We felt appalled by his behavior that had precipitated his ultimate demise, and we temporarily forgot about the educational opportunities that his physical body offered. He was dead, and half-dissected. We could not hurt him, and it would not have been appropriate to try. For the rest of the afternoon laboratory session, we did not particularly want to touch him, but we proceeded with our daily assignment anyway. By the end of the day, however, we did accomplish one goal: we came up with a nickname for the man.

"What a creep," one young woman in our group said. "I'm really disappointed in our cadaver!"

"I know," the other woman agreed. "That story is so awful."

"Maybe he got what was coming to him," shrugged the other young man in our group.

"Here we had gotten to appreciate this old man, letting us dissect him and all, and he turned out to have been an Ike Turner," I said, making reference to the only famous alleged wife abuser I could think of at the time. They laughed. "Hey, that's it! We should call him 'Ike'!"

The weeks continued. Our anger toward Ike subsided. We continued carving our way through the body's organs, identifying nerves and blood vessels along the way. We located more muscles, and the tendons that attach them to bones. We localized ligaments that held one bone in place with the next. We also progressively used more and more lime shaving cream. Ultimately, we had our last anatomy examination, which consisted of two parts. The first was a written test; the second part involved walking through the laboratory, where all of the cadavers had been set out on display.

Our instructors had placed numbered pins into different parts of each cadaver, and we were to identify each of the labeled structures. We all studied hard, and we all passed.

The course ended, and we were greatly relieved. We would eventually forget some of the memorized trivia, and we would not miss the formaldehyde. The next year, we put our knowledge of human anatomy to use, as we studied diseases in human pathology class. After that, we would encounter more internal organs, but those would be within living patients we would meet during hospital rotations in the latter half of medical school.

Once Gross Anatomy class was completed, I acknowledged to a few friends that I felt like a different person to some degree. Now that I had seen a human body completely, inside and out, I sometimes might look at people differently than before. No longer did I only look at a person's face or external physique. If I chose to, I might more vividly envision his internal structures, just from having seen another human dissected throughout his entirety. Of course, I do not choose to look at people this way often; indeed, the surface may sometimes be more than I want to see. Yet, in one sense, studying anatomy helped me gain a greater realization of what makes up a human being, and the experiences that then make a human life.

The more I learned about the amazingly functional bodies that compose our physical existences, the more respect, intrigue, and wonder I felt—and the less I could consider that our bodies may have randomly formed by sheer chance. Most organs have not just one function, but many. They multitask, and they do it beautifully, interconnected by nerves, vessels, and cells that carry all of the essential nutrients, minerals, hormones, and proteins that keep us functioning so smoothly and gracefully, for as long as they do. Gaining some understanding of our own anatomy and physiology can also allow us to feel greater awe, and connection, by examining the intricacies of equally complex nonhuman life forms as well.

The thermodynamic law of entropy states that matter, at least in a closed or isolated system, tends to arrange itself toward increasing disorder and disarray. The development of even a fascinatingly complex, single-celled organism is anything but disorder. When we try to contemplate the totality and detail within multi-celled, multi-organ, multisystem creatures with a psyche, the complexities can be overwhelming to fathom, and breathtaking to behold and experience. I hardly pretend to have any answers to the mysteries of life, and I may be completely wrong; but we have to consider that our composition and existence may be due to a brilliant combination of both exquisite framework and remarkable adaptation. This recognition may evoke awe and reverence, which can result in feelings of humility and gratitude. Perhaps those sentiments may then lead to satisfaction, or at least peace.

Despite the amazing strides in medical imaging, and science in general, what we do not know about our biological makeup surely still far exceeds what we do know. Consider some historical perspective: at the time of the writing of the United States Constitution—a document still revered for its wisdom and influence on governments and laws—common medical treatments included bloodletting, leeches, and avoiding ill humours of the night air. Construction of the Panama Canal—one of the greatest engineering feats of modern history—saw tens of thousands of deaths from malaria, typhoid, and yellow fever in the late 19th to early 20th centuries, until the knowledge become widespread that those diseases were transmitted by mosquitoes. World War I included the first major battles involving airplanes, yet there were still no antibiotics. Later during World War II, which brought the development and utilization of a new magnitude of destructive weapons, the relatively new penicillin was in such demand and scarce supply that urine was collected from people receiving penicillin, in order to recapture some of the excreted drug for injection into other patients.

We continually hear in the news that a particular food is good for us, until it is determined to be bad for us; until it is discovered to be more healthful after all.

In the second half of the 20th century, nations launched rockets into space around the time researchers concluded that repeatedly breathing tobacco smoke into one's lungs is, in fact, not a good idea. Practicing meditation as a natural, non-pharmacological means of relaxing and lowering blood pressure gained greater recognition in the 1970s, but was also criticized and viewed disdainfully by many western physicians, given that we had modern medicines to treat anxiety and hypertension.

Perhaps the most illustrative recent example of our limited medical understanding is that of the appendix. Many of us were taught in the past that the appendix serves no known purpose, and that perhaps it may be a nonfunctioning remnant from an earlier version of our primate ancestors. Yet the appendix is found in many species, and even in recent years, scientists have published intriguing studies about the function of the appendix, suggesting that its presence may be advantageous.

In addition to containing some lymphatic tissue and secreting some functional peptide hormones, the appendix serves as an important reservoir for the normal bacteria that live in our gut. We have many more bacteria in our digestive tract than we have cells in our bodies, and these bacteria serve an important symbiotic purpose, aiding not only digestion and nutrition, but affecting everything from our immune systems to even our moods. Time and further research may lead to a better understanding of this microbiome within us, not to mention its manipulation or alteration in modern civilization, including the burgeoning prebiotic and probiotic industry. Nevertheless, the data thus far is compelling: the microorganisms that harbor in the appendix may help repopulate the colon with beneficial bacteria once an infectious diarrhea has passed. Although the specifics are still under investigation, the appendix seems to serve a purpose—which is another way of saying it seems to be there for a reason. Again, studies reaching this logical explanation were published only within the last decade or so—around the same time that smartphones became ubiquitous, four decades after NASA sent astronauts to the moon. We are not talking about intricacies of the brain or spinal cord, which are clearly more complex and challenging to study. We are still learning to understand something so simple as the appendix: just a thin, tubular structure a few centimeters long that hangs off the first part of the large intestine.

Since taking my anatomy classes over thirty years ago, great strides have been made in medicine, from advances in imaging and diagnosis, to incredible new treatments. We may be on the cusp of game-changing developments in therapies tailored to people's genetic makeup, combined with greater access to shared human knowledge, augmented with artificial intelligence—but we still have a whole lot to learn.

We all clearly rely on our bodies more than we can ever fully appreciate. The workings of the body allow us to move, think, perform, experience, sense, and feel. Seeing Ike's body, bit by bit, helped heighten my awareness and understanding of the hardware required to live a human life.

Of course, Ike was already dead when I encountered him. Even had I been able to see the blood pumping through his veins, or the air expanding his living lungs, I would still have known virtually nothing about him, other than hearing second hand of his abusive domestic behavior that may have helped trigger his fatal heart attack. I had seen every bit of the physical mechanics left behind for examination: every organ, major nerve, and blood vessel that Ike had, from large bones, to tiny nerve branches and capillaries, even the contents of his last meal. Still, there had once been so much more that no longer met the eye.

In retrospect, I gained a new respect for Ike. By donating his body to science after his death, he gave four medical students an indelible look into part of what makes a human being. Because we knew next to nothing about him, he also indirectly illustrated that we are all composed of so much more than our physical makeup. His body was still intact the first day of anatomy class, yet his person was long gone. He lived his life and made an impact on others through his life's work and deeds. He also left a legacy that continues to provoke thought in me, years after my classmates and I put down our anatomy lab scalpels for the last time and continued with our studies.

Ike evidently had a very unflattering exit from this world. For all I know, he may have acted despicably on a regular basis. However, he left the gift of his body, allowing his entrails to be examined for the sake of teaching doctors who would continue to treat the living. We then continue our work, treating patients and teaching new students, who then continue on their journeys, trying to learn more and to perform better tomorrow than we do today.

Regardless of Ike's behavior just before his last breath, there was an element of goodness in the final gift of his body to medicine, for which I remain grateful. At the very least, his legacy reinforced the notion that a person is so much more than the sum of his parts.

THE JUDGE

The retired judge and I sat down to review his angiogram films, so that he could understand the severity of the blockage in the arteries supplying blood to his legs. He looked tired; his usual wit and charisma seemed a distant memory. He paused briefly before each sentence he uttered, as if to muster energy, and to review the accuracy of his statements before expressing them. The man was old before his time, in worse physical shape at age sixty-nine than most people who are older by a decade or more. His face had once been vivid, his eyes once quite expressive. Now they seemed dull and flat, despite the sense of humor and intelligence trapped inside.

Ten years beforehand he had survived a stroke. In fact he recovered enough to get by fairly well afterward, even returning to work in the courtroom for a few more years until he retired. Nevertheless, years of poorly controlled high blood pressure, obesity, diabetes, high cholesterol, and heavy smoking had taken their toll and left him with severely blocked arteries.

From resulting damage to his kidneys, he had been on permanent dialysis for two years. Dialysis kept him alive, doing what his kidneys no longer could, but it was definitely no equal substitute for healthy organs. Healthy kidneys continuously filter and smoothly regulate the body's water and electrolyte content, while dialysis shocks the system three times a week, with sudden adjustments in fluid and blood chemistry. The effect is often exhausting. This man now felt as if half his time was spent either undergoing dialysis, or recuperating from the treatment itself.

When he did feel well enough to interact with people, he could still charm them with humor, though he was physically weak.

He lived at an assisted living facility, where he was popular with staff and other residents. He could not walk far, but did enjoy going outside to sit on a bench and feel the warmth of the sun. One day while outside, he lost his balance kneeling down to feed a cat, fracturing his collar bone and elbow in the fall. Though he slowly began to recover from those injuries, he remained weak and a bit unsteady on his feet. Another day at the facility, he bumped his left shin on the foot pedal of a hospital bed and tore his skin.

After several months of ointment and bandage treatments, the open wound still had not healed. A specialist suspected artery blockage and recommended an angiogram of the man's legs, in order to assess his circulation. The angiogram showed complete blockage of the main artery to his left leg, starting from inside his pelvis and spanning all the way to the knee. Only small tributaries provided enough collateral blood flow to keep the leg alive. A complete blockage of an artery, even over a short distance, renders balloon angioplasty and stent placement unfeasible.

The only hope for improving blood flow to his leg might have been surgical, yet the distal arteries from the knee to his foot were also in such bad shape that surgery was considered too risky and likely to fail. Any incision on this man's leg would almost certainly not heal properly, and this would require an amputation high in the groin. Even the groin incision would require extensive surgical rerouting of blood vessels just to heal the amputation site. Such tampering with the arteries would shunt blood from the right leg to the left. This would then compromise blood flow to the right leg, which was also markedly diseased, just not so bad as the left. If the right leg blood supply were interrupted to help the left amputation stump heal, then there would be a high probability that the right leg might not receive adequate blood flow anymore, and would also probably have to be amputated. Risking a surgical procedure to save one left leg would therefore likely cost him both legs.

His left arm was already weakened by the stroke a decade ago. The arm's strength was further compromised by the dialysis shunt that had been surgically placed in his forearm, through which his blood flowed to the filtering machine and back again, three days a week. Living with no legs and one weak arm would mean an existence of very little independent mobility, in addition to dialysis and residual impairment from his stroke.

"In other words," he sighed, "medically speaking, I'm all f****d up."

Even in his state of serious decline, he remained somehow entertaining. Exhausted and nearly spent, he could still deliver a punch line in his gruff and sometimes acerbic manner.

He understood that having any surgery to attempt to restore blood flow to his legs would probably lead to a double amputation.

"I'm not gonna do that," he shook his head. "I don't want to end up like something from Kentucky Fried Chicken, with one leg buried over here, another leg over there...."

He declined surgery and enrolled in hospice.

This case was of particular interest to me. It fascinated me in part because this man had some of the most diseased arteries of all the angiogram studies I had ever seen. Yet I did not perform the x-ray study myself, or interpret it, as the man was not my patient. He was my father.

Very early in the process of drafting some of the stories for this collection, my dad experienced the physical decline described above. He even read the first couple of stories I wrote when I began thinking about writing this book, and I believe he liked what little he read. He knew that his prognosis was poor, and worsening. Yet he looked to me to help illustrate what his angiogram meant for him, in terms of treatment options, and what he could expect to happen. The doctor in me was intellectually curious, and I could help explain his condition to him. The son in me needed to ensure that we considered all reasonable avenues, before concluding that there was very little left that medical science could offer him, if he wanted to maintain any degree of residual physical independence and dignity.

Together we looked at the x-ray images. I drew diagrams and made reference to a plumbing system as a metaphor; he understood. Without an adequate blood supply, his shin ulcer could not heal. If it were to get infected, his body could not send enough blood to the area to fight the infection. The infection would then probably spread up the leg and enter his bloodstream. Without risking double amputation, the advances of modern time could not save him from potentially succumbing to gangrene. Medically he was near the end of his body's road. At some point, he would be faced with the decision of whether or not to continue dialysis.

Seeing a loved one's health decline, and having realistic expectations of one's eventual demise, are sad facts of life for all of us. Yet my father's case serves to remind me poignantly of a valuable lesson: there is a wealth of human being inside everyone's body— healthy or diseased—that no x-ray study can begin to visualize. We are made of so much more than the tissues and blood that compose our physical form. Direct visual inspection alone barely scratches the surface of understanding who we are, of what we are constructed, and of what we may be capable.

Dad's angiogram revealed the circulatory disease that contributed to his death. Imaging his vascular disease may also allow an observer to infer a few aspects of Dad's personality, by correctly assuming that he had been physically inactive and not particularly attentive to his health, given that the main causes of atherosclerosis include smoking, high cholesterol, uncontrolled hypertension and diabetes. Yet no one looking at his angiogram could imagine how those legs earlier in his life had spent so many weekend days slowly walking through woods while hunting, or how they helped him circle the bases in high school, when his passion was baseball.

If someone took an x-ray of his arm, they might see signs of an old, healed fracture from childhood. However, no radiologist could possibly envision how disappointed he was when the mildly limited range of motion resulting from that childhood fracture prevented him from receiving an ROTC scholarship after high school.

An x-ray of his neck would reveal pieces of shrapnel. By seeing his gender and age stamped on the corner of the film, a smart person might correctly deduce that the wound was inflicted during the Korean War. Yet no one looking just at shrapnel on his x-ray would know the details of the combat in which he was involved, or the pain and fear he must have felt from the injury that awarded him a Purple Heart.

If someone saw the CT scan of his head, they would see

signs of an old stroke in the right side of his brain. The observer could imagine that the patient must have been left with some neurological deficit. A neurologist reviewing the film might be a little more specific as to which body parts or functions were affected by the stroke, but only to a point. Even visualizing the human brain scientifically can be woefully limited in determining the impact of disease on one's mental and physical abilities.

No one could look at this head CT scan and appreciate that dad still had one of the keenest long-term memory capacities of anyone I have ever known. The CT pictures would not reveal how well he remembered people's names, nor the hundreds of humorous tales about people he knew. No picture of his brain could indicate how well Dad could captivate a room with a funny story, keeping people amused and engaged regardless of how many times they had heard the story before. His tales might reflect on growing up poor during the Depression, or recall a humorous incident from his courtroom. His stories gave him as much life as the blood in his veins. They revealed essential experiences and events that helped shape and demonstrate the person he was—but they could not be seen by the best radiologist in the world.

No one looking at Dad's head CT predicted that his stroke would leave him less hardened and reserved, and thus more capable of expressing feeling and showing emotion. A man who either did not believe in showing tears, or who once had few to shed, became more emotionally engaged and expressive after his stroke. My family is convinced that the change was not so much due to his newfound appreciation of being alive and functional, but rather to a genuine physical effect of the stroke. Rather than losing a center of speech or muscle control, he seemed to lose a center of reserve and inhibition. The result allowed him to open up and gave us all an opportunity to know and appreciate him better. In some ways, the years after his stroke were the most gratifying of his life. Although extremely ironic, losing a piece of his brain to stroke may have been one of the best things that ever happened to him, at least with regard to his personal relationships and appreciation for life.

These pivotal events and experiences throughout his life were fundamental in forming his mind, personality, and character. They were nearly as essential as the very brain cells that provided the biological framework for his thoughts and actions to exist in the first place. Both the anatomy and the life events served as building blocks, as key elements in forming the man.

For any individual, the exterior is visible to the human eye. Medical imaging may reveal someone's internal anatomy like a detailed road atlas, but there is still so much more to a person. Not being able to see concretely those elusive, intangible components of someone does not make those elements of a person less important, or less real. The inner character and personality—dare I say, the soul—of the human being may require the working physical body in order to be reflected and expressed. Yet perhaps recognizing the invisible essence that lies within each of us is an equally important lesson to learn from studying images of ourselves. We may be able to see more than ever before, but our visual skills still have plenty of shortcomings and limitations. There is so much more beneath the surface yet to be seen.

I try to remind myself that each patient who ever had an x-ray study performed may be every bit as complex as the next patient. Radiologists feel this when looking at x-rays of someone we know, but of course we usually do not know the person whose images we read. Sometimes we may ignore that each patient has his or her own stories, dreams, loved ones, and life experiences. A busy day at work may temporarily require all of one's energy to focus on anatomy and disease. When focused, we do our primary job helping patients, using technology to open them up without a scalpel. But focusing too narrowly on anatomy and disease may distance us from the deeper essence of the person being studied. I try to remember that each person is made up of so much more than bones and lungs, liver and pancreas. Every individual carries a unique combination of experiences, abilities, qualities, and shortcomings that make each of us human. The fact that I am unfamiliar with the depth of character and individuality not captured by the x-ray does not mean that these traits do not exist; they are present within each of us.

Recall some of the diagnoses made by imaging the people in these stories. Beyond tumors, strokes and infections, we detected everything from domestic violence to drug and alcohol abuse, even manifestations of mental illness. We diagnosed infertility for some, and unexpected pregnancy in another. In some people, we detected treatable conditions, while in others we found mortal illness beyond the reach of medical intervention. Foreign objects were discovered, each with its own story beyond the intrigue of these items being placed internally. We also saw serious complications from the hands of those who sought to heal.

These diagnoses could not have been made so easily, if at all, in past eras when modern imaging was unavailable. Who knows what people someday may be able to detect that currently eludes us.

We also glimpsed into the bodies and the lives of people who are very different, yet they all pass along the same thread of humanity. These people need not and cannot be defined by the findings on their images, because we are all more complex than any diagnosis. Some people let their spirits shine by finding resilience and strength to conquer weakness or vulnerability, refusing to be equated with their illnesses.

The power of radiology is incredible, and getting better all the time, yet there is still so much within people that remains concealed, yet to be uncovered and understood. Just because we cannot see it directly does not mean that it is not there.

Even with ever-improving scientific abilities to look within people, perhaps what most strongly makes us human is that which we cannot view, and in fact may never directly visualize. We see its elements reflected outwardly, and we intuitively believe that essence must exist. We may search with the human eye and come up empty-handed, but we inherently feel that there is more within. We can search with broader senses and discover understanding of the power, the spirit, and the potential within someone. We feel the impact as this force touches us and influences our thoughts and feelings. Its direct image may never be observed. Its true appearance may forever remain a mystery. But we may trust that it exists, as real as the brain within the head, the heart within the chest, or the smile upon the face.

GLOSSARY OF RADIOLOGICAL TERMS

Angiogram: a study that images blood vessels, i.e. arteries or veins.

CT (Computed Tomography; formerly Computed Axial Tomography, CAT or "CAT scan"): A technology that images the body using x-rays emitted from a large tube rotating around the patient. The images generated on a CT scan allow the radiologist to look at the patient one thin section at a time, like being able to look at each slice of bread in a loaf, or each card in a deck.

Mammogram: a special type of x-ray study designed to evaluate the breast, used to screen for breast cancer.

MRI (Magnetic Resonance Imaging): a technology that images the body using magnetic fields and radio waves instead of the ionizing radiation used in x-rays and CT scans.

Nuclear Medicine: a technology that images part of the body by having the patient receive a small dose of radioactivity internally by injection, swallowing, or breathing. Rather than expose a patient to an x-ray beam externally, nuclear medicine studies use an external camera that detects the radiation emitted from within the patient after the patient has received the dose.

PET (Positron Emission Tomography): a special type of nuclear medicine test, using radioactive isotopes that emit positrons (positively charged electrons) rather than the more common types of radiation emission used in other nuclear medicine studies.

Radiation: defined as the transport of energy through space. Radiation comes in different forms, including ionizing radiation (x-rays and gamma rays), and particulate radiation (electrons, positrons, alpha particles, neutrons). Like many things in life, it can be helpful or harmful, depending on how it is used.

Radiologist: a medical doctor specialized in interpreting imaging studies such as x-ray images (radiographs), ultrasound, CT, MRI, nuclear medicine, etc.

Radiology: the medical specialty of performing and interpreting studies that use energy such as x-rays, ultrasound waves, or magnetic waves to image the human body internally.

Radiation Oncology: the use of radiation to treat cancer. This is a medical specialty completely separate from radiology. Radiation oncology treatments require substantially higher doses of radiation than the amounts needed to take diagnostic x-ray images.

Technologist: an individual trained to perform x-ray, CT, MRI, nuclear medicine, or ultrasound studies to be interpreted by a radiologist. (Radiologists are highly dependent on and extremely grateful for the expertise of technologists!) The technologist is usually the first person, and often the only person, whom a patient may see when having a radiological study performed.

Ultrasound: a technology that images part of the body using high-frequency sound waves. These sound waves are at a frequency much too high to be heard by the human ear, hence the name ultrasound. Ultrasound studies might also be called sonograms, and an ultrasound technologist is also called a sonographer. An ultrasound performed on the heart is called an echocardiogram. An ultrasound performed on blood vessels may also be referred to as a Doppler study.

GLOSSARY OF MEDICAL TRAINING

Medical School: the curriculum of study by which a student attains a doctor of medicine degree, usually taking four years, completed after graduation from college.

Internship: the first year of supervised training after a doctor has completed medical school.

Residency: formal training within a chosen medical specialty after medical school. Decades ago, many doctors in training often lived at their teaching hospitals, hence the name "residents." Depending on the medical specialty, a residency usually takes three to five years to complete.

Fellowship: specialty training within a specific field of medicine, done after residency. Most fellowships are one to two years in duration, some longer.

ACKNOWLEDGEMENTS

Writing this book has been a labor of love and exploration. It has taken longer than I would have ever imagined, but that process has allowed the words on these pages to mature at their own pace.

I first express deep gratitude to the folks at Torchflame Books and Light Messages Publishing, for seeing potential and taking a chance on me. I also thank them for assigning me the superb editor Meghan Bowker, who was truly worth the wait.

Several fine authors deserve great thanks for their guidance and encouragement at earlier stages in development, including Bob Rosen, Julie Rold, Carolyn Jourdan, Frank Huyler, Doris Grumbach, and Jack Gardner. The organizational structure into themed sections was suggested by Mike Lesperance. I thank other friends for feedback on earlier drafts, in particular Joyce Love; and Jillian Poole, who gave me the kick I needed where I needed it the most.

I also acknowledge Patty Futrell and Teresa Lawler for transcription, and Melinda Byrns for reference assistance.

Thanks to my family for your support; and a special thanks to Yuta, for being a living example of patience, humility, positivity, and understanding.

REFERENCES

Chapter 1 (Images of Ourselves):

Brecher R, Brecher E. *The Rays: A History of Radiology in the United States and Canada.* Williams and Wilkins; 1969.

Doby T, Alker G. *Origins and Development of Medical Imaging.* Southern Illinois University Press; 1997.

Kevles B. *Naked to the Bone: Medical Imaging in the 20th Century.* Rutgers University Press; 1997.

Gunderman R. *X-Ray Vision: The Evolution of Medical Imaging and its Human Significance.* Oxford University Press; 2013.

Chapter 4 (People Like Us):

Harden V. *AIDS at 30: A History.* Dulles: Potomac Books; 2012.

Raja AS et al. Negative appendectomy rate in the era of CT: an 18-year perspective. *Radiology* 2010; 256:460-465.

Lahaye MJ et al. Mandatory imaging cuts costs and reduces the rate of unnecessary surgeries in the diagnostic work-up of patients suspected of having appendicitis. *European Radiology* (2015) 25:1464-1470.

Chapter 23 (Au Naturel):

Grobner T. Gadolinium—a Specific Trigger for the Development of Nephrogenic Fibrosing Dermopathy and Nephrogenic Systemic Fibrosis? *Nephrology Dialysis Transplantation* 2006; 21:1104-1108.

Marckmann P et al. Nephrogenic systemic fibrosis: suspected causative role of gadodiamide used for contrast-enhanced magnetic resonance imaging. *Journal of the American Society of Nephrology* 2006; 17:2359-2362.

Rydahl, C, Thomsen, HS, Marckman, P. High prevalence of nephrogenic systemic fibrosis in chronic renal failure patients exposed to gadodiamide, a Gadolinium (Gd)- containing magnetic resonance contrast agent. *Investigative Radiology* 2008; 43:141-144.

Thomsen, HS. Nephrogenic systemic fibrosis: a serious adverse reaction to gadolinium 1997-2006-2016. *Acta Radiologica* 2016, Vol. 57(5) 515-520 (Part 1) and 57(6) 643-648 (Part 2).

Pullicino R et al. A Review of the Current Evidence on Gadolinium Deposition in the Brain. *Clinical Neuroradiology* (2018) 28:159-169.

Ramalho M et al. Gadolinium Retention and Toxicity—An Update. *Advances in Chronic Kidney Disease* 2017; 24(3):138-146.

Chapter 24 (Hard to Swallow):

Kraeft JJ, Uppot RN, Heffess AM. Imaging Findings in Eating Disorders. *AJR* 2013; 200:W328-W335.

Riddlesberger MM, Cohen HL, Glick PL. The swallowed toothbrush: A Radiographic Clue of Bulimia. *Pediatric Radiology* 1991: 21(4):262-4.

Chapter 27 (Inside Out):

Courcoulas AP et al. Seven-Year Weight Trajectories and Health Outcomes in the Longitudinal Assessment of Bariatric Surgery (LABS) Study. *JAMA Surgery* 2018; 153(5): 427-434

Aminian A et al. Association of Metabolic Surgery with Major Adverse Cardiovascular Outcomes in Patients with Type 2 Diabetes and Obesity. *JAMA* 2019; 322(13): 1271-1282.

Jakobsen GS et al. Association of Bariatric Surgery vs Medical Obesity Treatment with Long-term Medical Complications and Obesity-Related Comorbidities. *JAMA* 2018; 319(3): 291-301.

Schauer PR et al. Bariatric Surgery versus Intensive Medical Therapy for Diabetes 5-year outcomes. *New England Journal of Medicine* 2017; 376:641-51.

Chapter 33 (Ike):

McNeill WH. *Plagues and Peoples*. Anchor; 1976.

McCullough D. *The Path Between the Seas*. Simon and Schuster; 1978.

Adams DP. Wartime Bureaucracy and Penicillin Allocation: The Committee on Chemotherapeutic and Other Agents, 1942-44. *Journal of the History of Medicine and Allied Sciences*, 1989 Vol. 44, No. 2, 196-217.

Bollinger R, et al. Biofilms in the large bowel suggest an apparent function of the human vermiform appendix. *Journal of Theoretical Biology* 2007; 249(4):826-831.

Ansaloni L, Catena F, Pinna AD. What is the function of the human vermiform appendix? Evolution-based surgery: a new perspective in the Darwinian year 2009. *European Surgical Research* 2009;43(2):67-71.

Merchant R et al. Association Between Appendectomy and Clostridium Difficile Infection. *Journal of Clinical Medicine Research* 2011; 4(1):17-19.

Laurin M, Everett ML, Parker W. The Cecal Appendix: One More Immune Component with a Function Disturbed by Post-Industrial Culture. *The Anatomical Record* April 2011, Vol. 294(4): 567-579.

Yong FA et al. Appendectomy: a risk factor for colectomy in patients with Clostridium difficile. *The American Journal of Surgery*, 2015 Vol. 209 (3), 532-535.

ABOUT THE AUTHOR

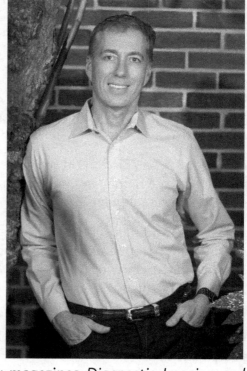

Cullen Ruff, MD, is a radiologist in private practice, and an associate professor at the Virginia Commonwealth University campus in Fairfax, VA, where he has received awards teaching medical students.

Chapters from *Looking Within* have appeared in *Radiology Today* and *UU World* magazines, and in 2019, Ruff won a Washington, DC *Moth* story slam narrating a chapter from *Looking Within*.

The author has published in online forums *Univadis, Doximity, KevinMD, ImagingBiz, XrayVsn,* and *Waiting Room*; and radiology magazines *Diagnostic Imaging and Radiology Business Journal*, in addition to scientific journal articles. Ruff is a Fellow of the American College of Radiology.

www.cullenruff.com

CPSIA information can be obtained
at www.ICGtesting.com
Printed in the USA
LVHW011132171220
674417LV00004B/595